INSTINCTIVE
BIRTHING

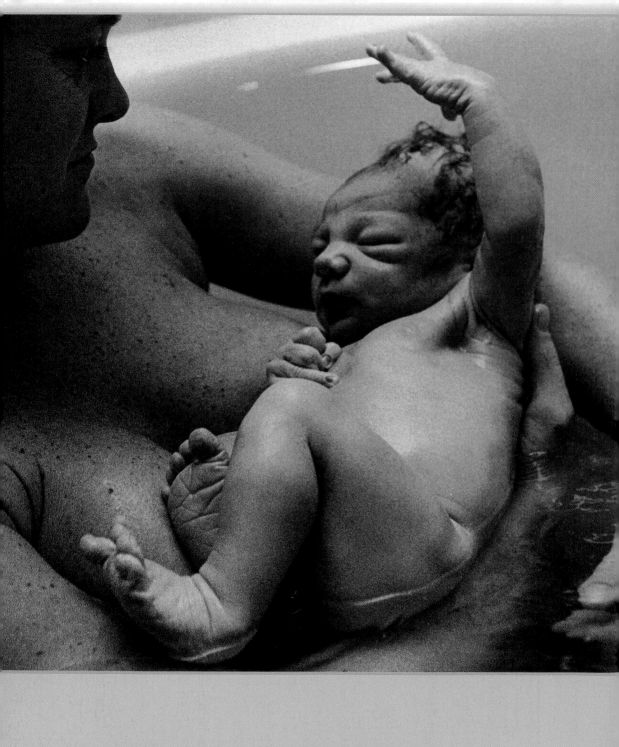

INSTINCTIVE
BIRTHING
Heeding your inner voice

VAL CLARKE

with Helen Massay-Alstrom

CARROLL & BROWN PUBLISHERS LIMITED

To all "my" mothers whose experiences made me the midwife I am today

This edition published in 2005 in the United Kingdom by

Carroll & Brown Publishers Limited
20 Lonsdale Road, London NW6 6RD

Text © Val Clarke 2005
Compilation © Carroll & Brown Limited 2005

A CIP catalogue record for this book is available from the British Library.

ISBN 1-904760-02-3

10 9 8 7 6 5 4 3 2 1

Reproduced by RDC, Malaysia
Printed and bound in Spain by Bookprint, S.L., Barcelona

CONTENTS

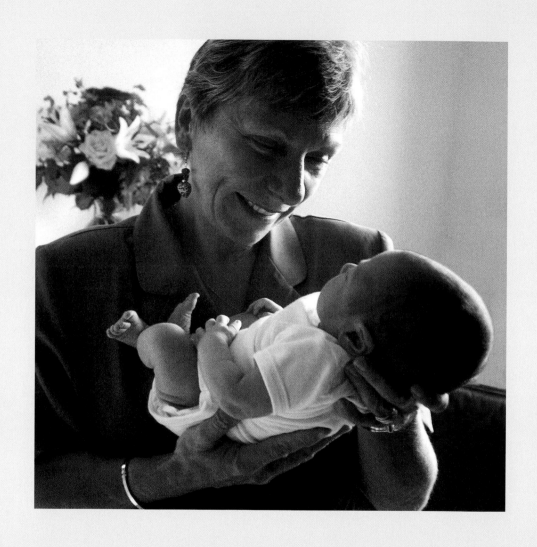

FOREWORD
by Sheila Kitzinger

Here is the wise reassuring voice of an experienced midwife who believes that women should be enabled to trust their instincts in pregnancy, birth and beyond. She cites many examples of birth experiences in which she and the mother working together have trusted their gut feeling and describes how this has helped birth be natural and unforced, or in some cases has resulted in the decision to go to hospital when it turned out that this level of care was needed.

She urges women to question whether the wide range of screening tests in pregnancy and the proliferation of technology in childbirth are really helpful and to "listen" to their bodies and their babies still in the womb.

There has been heavy emphasis in recent government and midwifery publications on informed choice. That is good. Yet perhaps the importance of inner confidence in one's birthing body has been overlooked.

Val is the skilled, warm midwife friend every woman might wish she could have.

Having a child is a wonderful gift. If you are already pregnant, your miracle has begun, and you have already embarked on an amazing relationship. Loving your child will be a very personal emotion, a feeling that is hard to describe. Words such as eternal, unconditional, and completely fulfilling spring to mind but to choose just a single word seems to underestimate the intensity of such incredible love. I feel an overwhelming sense of happiness when I see any woman who is pregnant; it reminds me of all my joy and fulfilment as a mother of four boys, but I also anticipate the wonderful moments this woman is about to encounter.

As a midwife of 25 years' standing, I have been thinking about this book for at least half this time. I wanted to write a book that would equip pregnant women with insight and inspiration: insight that would help them to understand what they are about to experience, so they could ask the right questions of caregivers, and become confident and empowered mothers from the moment they discovered a baby inside; inspiration that would give them the confidence to explore some of the available options, and to help them to work in tandem with mind and body to find some of the answers.

In many ways having a baby sounds so simple, yet for those of you who have already encountered challenges conceiving a child, you will already appreciate that it is not as simple as it seems. No two women are exactly the same, and no two birthing experiences either. But no matter the differences, I believe that every pregnancy and birth is special, and that every woman has the right to enjoy her experience for what it is, in spite of what she may deem to be standard or the norm.

Every woman hopes to have a wonderful birth and a perfect baby. While this book cannot influence the latter, I sincerely hope that it helps you to achieve a successful birth, which will be the basis for your new role as a successful mother. Your experience will also mould your perception of the process, and may influence the approach you take towards future births.

As a midwife, my ethos has always been to practice instinctively and holistically, creating a trusting relationship with women, which I hope paves the way for a positive birthing experience. I want mothers to feel that they have had the opportunity to work with their bodies – knowing that they and their babies were safe – and that their best interests were considered, rather than entering labour in fear and trepidation. Their (and my) best result is to experience childbirth in the way they envisaged, surrounded by people they know, trust and love. At the very least, a woman should understand all the options available, and be able to make the best of any unforeseen situation in an informed manner, with the proviso that nature will have the last word.

Every woman's idea of a perfect birth will be different though nature and circumstance play a huge part in dictating what actually happens. In many respects, they will dictate the outcome of your birthing experience. But it is just as possible for a woman to have an emergency caesarean and feel she has had a wonderful birth as it is for a woman who decides to have her baby at home with her older children playing around her! The key is not what happened, but that you were able to participate in the decisions taken, using the knowledge available at the time, and made an informed choice. In other words, you can look back on the birth and understand what happened, why it happened, and feel that you were a part of the decision-making process. Only you can judge what is your perfect birth; my role in this book is not to challenge your beliefs, but to help you to ask the right questions and make the choices that are right for you.

Gathering information and asking questions is an important aspect of parenting, and one that starts as soon as you find out you are pregnant. One particular aspect of pregnancy and childbirth that has transformed modern-day maternity care is technology. We have witnessed major advances in obstetric care, and

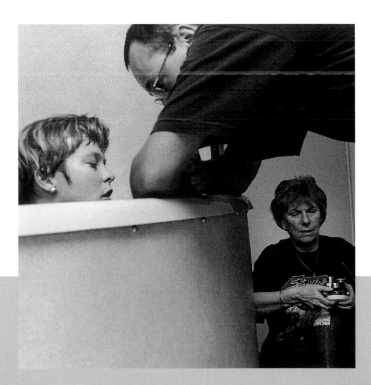

many women owe their lives to advanced technological procedures. However, there can be a tendency to use technology routinely and at the expense of less invasive care. While I wholly applaud technology and accept that further advances will be made, it is important to understand its use and purpose in order to feel comfortable that it is in your, and your baby's, best interest.

One of the objectives of this book is to help you to achieve your ideal birth whether you choose to use private or state-funded care. Generally speaking, the private sector is able to offer greater time for discussion and a more personal approach to care. In many countries, the state-funded sector is heavily stretched in terms of financial resources and personnel, which means time for care and choice of care become critical issues.

Having worked in both the independent and state-funded sector, I have seen the pros and cons of each. I always tried to apply my philosophy of care whether I was working in the state or private sector. While this book is certainly not a sales pitch for independent midwifery, as this may or may not be practically or financially viable for many people, the independent sector does provide a service that is more tailored to the individual. I found that birthing outcomes in the private sector were generally better, as women had a one-to-one relationship with their midwives and more confidence in themselves and their instincts.

That said, I know many women who experienced wonderful births within the state system. I do believe you can make the system work for you. This book will help you to find out what is on offer, and will explain how it is within your power to overcome some of the shortfalls you may encounter.

Much parental responsibility involves making decisions on behalf of our offspring. Some decisions are easier to make than others, and each of us has a different way of finding the right answer. Pregnancy and childbirth are no exceptions; you'll be amazed at the number of decisions you will be asked to make even before your child is born.

When it comes to decision-making, there is one aspect of our lives that I feel is gradually being eroded. That is our inner voice, our instinct. Looking back over the years, I can see how women have come to depend less and less on their feminine instincts. Substantial prenatal care, increased rates of intervention, and more advanced technology have created an environment that demands very little input from a woman's basic instinct. While I do acknowledge that infant mortality rates have decreased substantially, it saddens me that pregnancy is no longer a sacred time for women to listen to their bodies and heed the information with which they were equipped since birth.

There is, however, a way to play a larger part in the proceedings, and the decisive factor is confidence. If you are aware of the facts and are in tune with your needs – be that at a mental or physical level – you will be more in control. If you are aware of your instincts, and are able to trust what your mind is telling you, you will feel stronger about decisions being made. I have seen a great deal of instinctive behaviour over the years. I wanted to share with you the value that it can bring. When all else fails, instinct will usually be the one source that you can turn to for an answer.

Being pregnant in the 21st century is a serious affair, as you will no doubt discover when you go to the bookshop! There is a wealth of books available on all aspects of pregnancy and birth, ranging from the medical to practical to the comical. In many ways you are in a vulnerable position, and the content of your reading material may make a significant impression on your approach to childbirth. This book is not an A to Z of what to expect when you are pregnant. Its objective is to equip you mentally and emotionally for those moments over the proceeding months when you are not sure of what is happening, or for what purpose. I hope my book helps you to understand what is available, and to assess its relevance to your situation. All you can ever expect to do is what is right and on offer at the time. Even if the services available are not perfect, they certainly can be exploited in your best interest.

I hope you have caught some of the passion and inspiration I want so desperately to share with you. The more births I see, the more I am convinced that we can have a say in what happens, and there are ways to influence outcome. Your mind is very powerful; if you equip it with knowledge and awareness, it will help direct you towards the right decision. Your body is another strong ally, and was designed to give birth. Be confident and, most importantly, enjoy your pregnancy and birth experience.

Note: references to the baby throughout this book will be in the masculine and those to midwives in the feminine. This is not meant to stereotype or generalize, but is a consistent way to refer to those people in a way that is most familiar to me, as a female midwife and the mother of four boys!

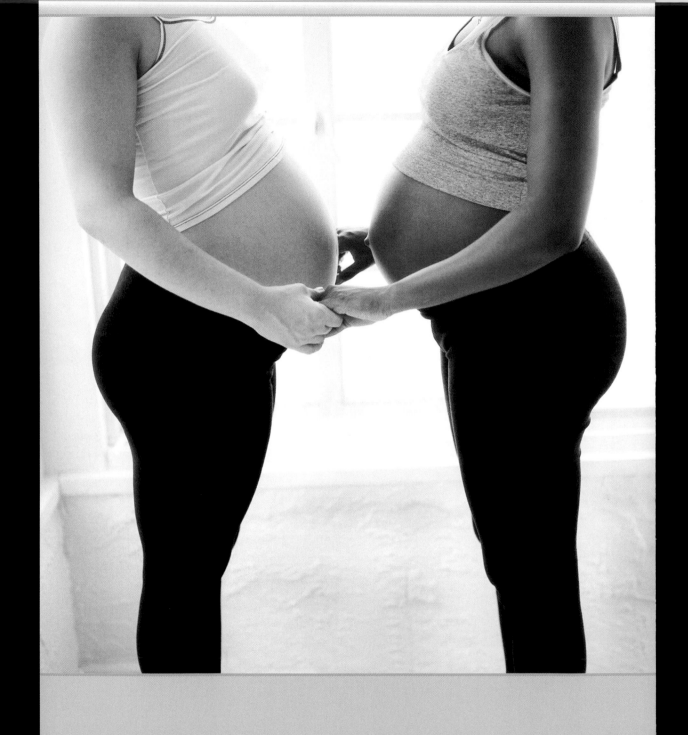

CHAPTER 1
21st-century Pregnancy

21ST-CENTURY PREGNANCY

Not so very long ago, a couple could depend on their extended families for help and protection throughout pregnancy, during childbirth, and in the weeks afterwards. These days, however, families tend to be smaller in size and individual members don't interact as much as they once did. Now, it's much more common for people to move to new areas and even new countries in search of employment opportunities and/or a different quality of life and, although we have greater means of communicating at speed and low cost, we usually don't see members of our extended families on a daily basis, and we no longer rely on their physical presence and help as we once did. This has had an interesting impact on pregnant women and new mothers, who are forced to be more self-reliant than their predecessors.

BRAVE "NEW" WOMEN

As well as the family unit, women, too, have changed radically over the last century. Not that long ago, most women's expectations were to complete their education, which was often limited; get married and have babies. Once married, women were expected to manage a household and all its related chores, such as shopping, cooking, cleaning, mending and making. A woman would give birth to her children, often at home, and while they were young, spend all day in their company, nurturing them. This was what society expected and, in some circles, imposed upon women. Family influence was great, and women relied on the experience and knowledge of mothers and grandmothers in taking care of their homes and children. Women's instincts – particularly as related to domestic matters and especially in pregnancy and childbirth – prevailed within the framework of this extended family.

But the 20th century brought numerous opportunities for women to play a greater role in the external world, particularly of business and politics. More and more women started to pursue career options, partly for financial reasons but also to make greater use of their intellectual abilities. Even where women only worked part time, it allowed them some entry into the outside world and interrupted the tradition of their staying at home full time. This impacted significantly on society; the relationship between men and women that had existed for as long as people could remember, began to change. Instead of men being the sole providers, women were contributing to household expenses and starting to express a view on how income was spent. And, they also started to want their spouses to share domestic chores and responsibilities.

Today, it is expected that many women will be educated to graduate level and that they will not rush into having children. Women who have spent the best part of sixteen years studying don't relish the idea of relinquishing all the knowledge and experience they've acquired in order to start having babies right away. Moreover, during their education or training, most will live away from home, and once they graduate, their

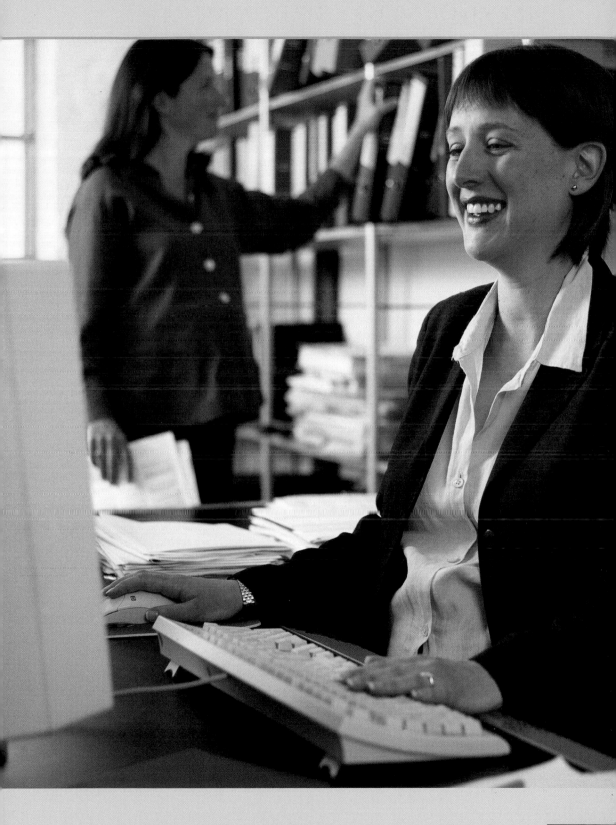

goal is to get a paid job that will support a continuing independent life, and hopefully, meet their financial commitments. While student debt may entice some women back home, most will opt not to return to the family nest once their education and training is complete. The majority will pursue a career path of some kind.

Because women now wield greater financial and political power, this has transformed the way society values them. Today, how well a woman sews, cooks or knits, is less admired than her earning power, strength and tenacity, and ability to retain her youthful appearance. Women run marathons, set up and direct companies, and some even become prime ministers. In most areas, the gap between men and women is closing every day and, with the exception of some physical constraints, the sexes are competing on a fairly level footing. Today's women must juggle priorities day in day out and keep the basic wheel of society well oiled; it's not surprising then that, in general, they have become independent and self-sufficient, a state of mind and being that can be at odds with the mechanisms and demands of pregnancy.

EXERCISING CONTROL

Having witnessed a great many pregnancies and births, I am aware of just how beautiful and marvellous those experiences can be. Being at the centre of a process in which a few cells develop into a tiny fetus and then into a responsive human baby, is something most women find miraculous. And in experiencing the intense joy and fulfilment that a baby brings both his parents, a woman partakes of life's sublime achievement.

But pregnancy and childbirth are not always supremely satisfying experiences. They sometimes bring sorrow. Having experienced the loss of a baby, both personally and through my work, I am also well aware of the pain and anguish that can accompany pregnancy and birth. Nor does the miracle of pregnancy always manifest. The majority of couples, thankfully, are able to conceive readily and naturally, but some need assistance, and there are those fated never to have babies at all. As much as we may try to arrange the arrival of our children, there seem to be certain forces outside our control, and these may prevail in the end.

These days the uncertainty of pregnancy seems a particularly hard message to deliver, as many women now expect to be able to plan a pregnancy and have a certain level of control over the timing of their conceptions, and assisted conception techniques have advanced significantly, helping many of those who do not find conceiving a baby as easy as they had imagined.

Our lives are much more scheduled than ever they were in the past and, for some women, pregnancy is merely another event that needs to be a given a slot in the diary. Although there are plenty of stories of unexpected pregnancies, teenage "mistakes" and fertility problems – which may contradict this statement – the ability to pinpoint the exact time in your life when you will have a baby has never been easier. Contraception has facilitated the timing of one's babies tremendously. Women taking the contraceptive pill can put their fertility on hold for a set period of time and be almost one hundred percent certain that they won't become pregnant. Since many women start taking the pill as soon as they begin a sexual relationship, and continue to take it while at college, throughout their early career, and until they are in a settled relationship and the prospect of parenthood becomes more appealing, this could mean taking the pill for between two and 20 years.

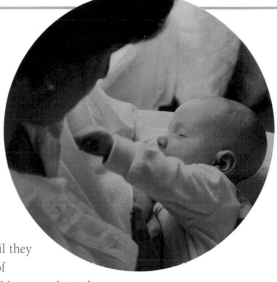

"Elderly primigravidae" or women having first babies at a relatively late age are a sign of our times. Better antenatal care has ensured safer deliveries and healthier babies.

Ovulation kits allow you to check each month for the existence of luteinizing hormone, and thus ascertain whether or not you are ovulating. Using this simple method, it is possible to increase the chances of either avoiding an unwanted pregnancy or encouraging one that is desired. Blood tests and ultrasonography can determine the hormone balance within the body, whether a woman has ovulated, and the general state of her reproductive system. IVF (In Vitro Fertilization) has created opportunities for people with fertility problems to conceive a child (or several children!) and overcome many barriers imposed by nature.

All these aids have helped us to become more aware of what is happening inside our bodies, to provide us with an opportunity to take control of our fertility clock, and to govern, to a certain extent, when we will start a family.

AGE CONSIDERATIONS

Childbearing trends have moved with the times and undergone quite a significant shift over recent decades. Because most couples require two incomes to establish a household, and most women expect to pursue some kind of career after completing their education, babies tend to be something we think about only after we've established ourselves financially and professionally. Today, a woman's priorities are finding a well-paying job, and getting her foot on the housing ladder. Once these are in place, she can begin to think seriously about relationships and family life. This has naturally led to a tendency to have children later than our mothers and grandmothers did.

The importance of age in pregnancy can't be ignored; we are bumping up against the boundaries of fertility by delaying childbearing until our less fertile years.

While in human terms, 30 to 40 is still very young (and getting younger every day!), as regards fertility, this is really quite old. A woman's fertility is at her greatest in her early twenties and, in spite of all our efforts to prolong human life, we have not been able to widen the fertility window significantly.

Even if you become pregnant at an "advanced" age (between 30 and 45), there are well-documented risks associated with older mothers. Older mothers have a much greater chance of producing children with Down syndrome, and experiencing pregnancy-related hypertension, long and/or difficult labours, and forceps deliveries or caesarean sections. Yet the simple fact is that today many of us are just not ready to have children in our twenties. The timing of children is one of those complex matters where there is a conflict between what nature intended for our bodies and the progressive evolution of the human mind.

I feel it is a midwife's duty to listen intently to what every expectant mother says about her feelings, her hopes and her fears. This is even more important when there are potentially greater risk factors. A mother at risk often feels that her instinctive voice is being ignored and, very often, this is true.

"AT-RISK" MOTHERS

One of the recurring messages of this book is the role a midwife can play throughout the months of pregnancy and during birth. One vital aspect is the provision of information, particularly if a woman is regarded by "the system" as a potential risk. An expectant mother of whatever age needs to be equipped very early on in her pregnancy with information on the experience ahead, both as to what is happening within her body and how she'll be treated within the healthcare system. When a woman is offered informed choice, she and her baby can be cared for as any normal healthy mother-to-be, unless nature deems otherwise. She begins to feel special and that her voice is being heard at all times.

My experience with pregnant mothers has been that in sharing my knowledge of what happens during pregnancy and birth – both inside and out – these mothers become emotionally stronger and their instinctive awareness increases. The result is that, unless there is a genetic or congenital problem, women who are older or otherwise at risk, will approach pregnancy, labour and birth with amazing strength and determination, which will have a favourable effect on the eventual outcome. This also applies to mothers who may be very young and those who may have learning difficulties. In both these situations, the type of care provided by a midwife requires additional consideration, as these pregnancies often involve quite complex and sensitive issues. However, the fact that a woman is preparing to have a baby remains unchanged even if she is 15; a teenager will

Having reluctantly terminated an untimely pregnancy several years before, Marcia and her partner were at last keen to become parents. Sadly, Marcia was told that she was, in fact, menopausal, and could no longer become pregnant naturally. The news, although devastating, soon became the beginning of another opportunity for this couple – the possibility of assisted conception. After exploring several options, egg donation became their chosen route. This procedure is similar to IVF but instead of the mother's egg (ovum) being used, a donor egg is obtained and fertilized by the partner's sperm and then implanted into the woman's womb. Happily, Marcia and her partner were lucky first time around. Marcia advanced well in her uncomplicated pregnancy. Interestingly, it was her partner who had difficulty in accepting Marcia's changing situation. The dynamic businesswoman whom he had fallen in love with was slowly becoming distinctly maternal in shape and emotions. Believing very strongly that the thoughts and feelings of pregnant partners should be explored, I gave him plenty of time and opportunity to talk about the situation. Becoming a father can often be a daunting proposal for men already burdened by the increasing responsibilities of our present day and age. Marcia's partner appreciated our informal chats, and became increasingly supportive of her growing pregnancy needs. Marcia birthed a beautiful baby girl without complication at her chosen place – the nearest hospital. Breastfeeding, too, was successfully established after a few weeks.

go through many of the same experiences as a woman in her twenties or thirties. Although the essence of this book is directed at a standard pregnancy, the experiences encountered by a woman who is pregnant will be similar whatever her situation.

WORK AND OTHER COMMITMENTS

When it comes to pregnancy and childbirth, women often expect and are expected to be superwomen. They are acclaimed for holding the fort at home, working as much as possible, and ignoring any pain or fatigue their bodies may be experiencing. The problem is that, while our minds have changed and adopted more of a male's approach to life, we have a female's body, and that body still requires the same level of rest and nurture during a pregnancy as it did when we were pretty much confined to home.

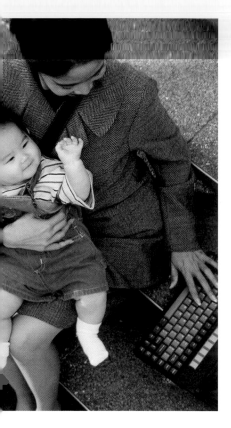

It's important that companies put into place more flexible working, allowing employees to find a more sustainable balance between their professional and personal lives.

In many workplaces, the pressures on mothers-to-be generally continue unabated. They strive to fulfil their responsibilities with stoic determination until they are able – at long last – to start their maternity leaves. Today's pregnant women usually expect to work for as long as possible. Sadly, legislation is painfully slow in recognizing that our future is our babies, and financial assistance is grossly compromised. This was never meant to be, but we have to accept it as part of the change in social structure. Most expectant mothers feel they need to work to achieve their financial objectives and maintain their lifestyles. Is this what's really best for mother and baby? Where have we gone wrong? Our obsession with financial gain and material possessions has led us to believe that what was good enough for our parents is no longer sufficient for us, yet I wonder if we are really any happier then they were or whether we just have access to more choice – choice at the expense of instinct and the unique ability of a mother to nurture her child for at least the first year of his life.

The reality of being a couple today is that once two people are in some kind of long-term relationship, the basis for their joint financial expectations and investments will be one of a dual income. Mortgages will be supported by two salaries and very little thought is given to the possibility of living on one salary – or of abandoning one career – at a time in the future.

Of course I am not suggesting that women revert to mid-twentieth century life and earlier, and spend all day sewing, caring for children and waiting for their husbands to return home, but I do feel there is a better way of balancing work and home life. Money will mean nothing to your baby; your time and love will be everything. The greater the balance you strike between your financial aspirations and the emotional needs of your baby, the more you will relish the privilege of parenthood. Furthermore, your child will thrive and benefit from the emotional foundation that you provide in his early years. A nursery, child minder, or nanny may be able to care for and oversee the development of your child, but real emotional nurturing comes from the family and, most importantly, from the mother.

Maybe we have cultivated a belief that parenthood should not disturb the status quo too much and that pre-baby life should resume as soon as possible after the birth. If this is the case, I would suggest we have also forgotten the way in which a child and his parents bond and, as a result, many women will find themselves grossly unprepared for the battle of the instincts.

THE CHANGING FAMILY UNIT

Another factor that contributes to delayed pregnancies is the disintegration of the extended family unit. It is no longer likely that a mother-to-be will be nurtured in the bosom of her family before and after her baby has arrived. She is much more likely to rely on herself and her partner for support, rather than her family. In many cases, a woman deems that her continuing control and independence must remain intact, as anything else would be a sign of weakness.

"For many women, carrying a child, being aware of the pulse of a new life pulsating within them, is the catalyst for re-evaluating their place in the world. It becomes a time to review priorities and decide the extent to which they will allow the conventions and values of the world at large to influence their personal behaviour."

Alternative Therapies for Pregnancy and Birth by Pat Thomas

Today's first-time parents feel a sense of failure if they are unable to cope with the demands of parenthood. They often perceive childbearing as a huge responsibility combined with a loss of freedom – both true to some extent. The irony is that the fundamental transformation that we experience in becoming parents is an aspect of life we were never meant to shoulder alone, but one for which support could be sought from parents, grandparents and the others in the extended family.

Some years ago, Sally and Andrew, a highly respected professional couple, retained me as their midwife. Sally, aged 40 at the time, confessed that it had taken her and Andrew seventeen years to harmonize their desire to have a baby. She explained that when one had felt the time had been right for parenthood, the other hadn't agreed, and that they'd respected each other's wishes as professionals. This first pregnancy went well and three years later, when Sally was 43, they had another little boy. Sally spent a year at home with each of her babies and then returned to her profession in a part-time capacity.

SINGLE MOTHERS

While in the past, an "unwed" mother was a source of scandal, today women increasingly undertake to have a baby on their own – whether because they feel they can afford to or because they become pregnant while in a relationship that ends when they are pregnant. In my experience, a fortunate single mother is one suppported by a loving family, her decision-making made easier as to when, where, and how she will birth her baby. And, in the case of a young mother years away from completing her education, whether she will keep her baby.

Single mothers, above all expectant women, need tender, loving, care. While instinctively fiercely protective of their unborn babies, they often become victims of the conveyor belt system of birthing. Such mothers find it almost impossible to labour and birth their babies as their instinct tells them. The support and reassurance they would look for in a partner simply doesn't exist – unless they are very fortunate with their friends and family. Yet such women often are very determined.

✳ Alice, a very attractive high-flying businesswoman, earned a substantial salary, owned a beautiful home, and had an on-and-off boyfriend, Carl. She had everything that life could offer except a baby. Although neither Alice nor Carl wanted to make a permanent commitment, Alice was desperate for a child and Carl had agreed to father one. Apart from some nausea in the early weeks, Alice had a trouble-free pregnancy, during which she celebrated her 46th birthday. Plans were made for Alice to birth her baby at home. Having had chorionic villus sampling, she knew she was having a daughter and was so excited at the prospect of becoming a mother, she positively bloomed as the birth drew near. Labour began spontaneously just beyond the "due" date and advanced slowly but without complication. Alice coped brilliantly with strength and acquired wisdom and tenacity, finally birthing a beautiful 8½ lb. girl. At six weeks, breastfeeding was well established and she was feeling "deeply fulfilled". I said goodbye but still hear from her each Christmas, and she has never once regretted her decision to become a single mother.

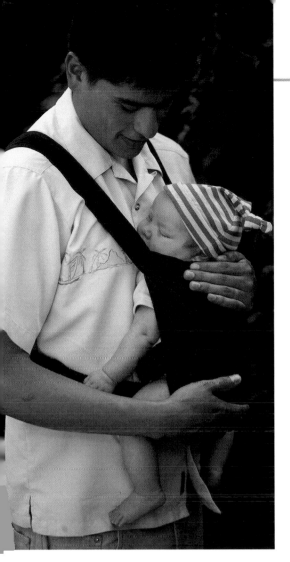

Increasing numbers of men are backing away from the demands of certain careers and seeking the chance to spend quality time with their children.

THE EFFECTS OF PREGNANCY ON A MAN

Over the last thirty years, the role of men in society also has undergone significant change. Men are increasingly comfortable with women in the workplace, partly because legislation requires it, and partly because they can see the value that a woman brings to the business, and how this can be complementary to that provided by a man. Because men and women tend to work in different ways, effective team-working is usually achieved by a blend of the sexes. In terms of family life, women now play a greater role in financial decisions, among other areas, while men are participating more actively in the running of their households, and in the care of their children. It is becoming more and more acceptable for a man to openly provide his family with the same level of commitment that he gives to his job, and many companies are endeavouring to support this through more flexible working and social policies, allowing employees to find a more sustainable balance between their professional and personal lives.

In view of this, it is only natural that men are taking more of an interest in pregnancy, the forerunner to family life. There are many ways in which a man can be involved in pregnancy. I find it really wonderful to see a man proud of his pregnant wife, and to hear him discuss the progress she is making in her pregnancy, the development of their baby, and their plans for the birth. Many men buy books

A man who is educated about pregnancy and birth is better able to support his partner through childbirth and to help her achieve as happy and successful an experience as possible.

Katy was happily pregnant for the first time. However, as her healthy pregnancy advanced, she confided to me that Steven, her partner, was becoming more and more withdrawn and refusing to discuss the forthcoming event – even though the decision to become pregnant had been a joint one. On the surface, there were no obvious reasons for Steven's behaviour but he did decline my invitations to join Katy and me when we met for antenatal appointments. Shortly before the birth, Steven returned to his parental home. Did he do so because "his inner child" had not been recognized while he was growing into adulthood or did he feel overwhelmed by increasing financial demands and the prospect of becoming "chief cook and bottle washer" once the baby was born? Happily, Steven did attend the birth of his son and eventually was reunited with Katy and their newborn.

(some targeted directly at them), obtain information from the Internet, and take a very active role in attending hospital appointments, scans and antenatal classes. As many women want their partners to be birth partners as well, a woman can only be encouraged when she sees her partner keen to confront the birthing experience as well-equipped with knowledge and information as she is.

In spite of acquiring knowledge, and being involved in planning the pregnancy and birth, many fathers-to-be experience an internal struggle with the prospect. Once a viable pregnancy has been confirmed and the early euphoria starts to abate, reality dawns. Although many men want to enjoy the activities surrounding pregnancy and the birth of their babies, few are afforded the time or opportunity to explore and voice their feelings, be they positive or negative. Becoming a father in this day and age demands so much that it is quite natural for a man to become completely overwhelmed with the expectations thrust upon him. Instinctively he wants to provide the safest environment for the woman who is carrying his baby. Unfortunately, many external factors play a part in eroding those instinctive feelings. Chief among them is that parenthood has become so commercialized that many men are unable to focus on anything other than the impending financial commitment. With pressure to possess all the "must-haves", all a man can envisage is the financial outlay spiralling upwards, possibly out of control. So what then of the newly pregnant father and his ability to cope with the harsh reality he faces?

Nature never intended life and living to be as potentially complicated as it is today. Having a baby was supposed to be a simple act of love whereby instinctive feelings led a loving couple to desire that their union bore fruit. Nature's expectation for a couple was that they be nurtured within the bosom of their extended family, thus enabling the expectant father to provide a safe shelter, while his wife was free to rest, eat, sleep and care for the child within.

Alas, for most men, pregnancy and birth are definitely not as nature intended.

It is difficult for a man to provide a safe and secure haven for his pregnant partner when the extended family is in steady decline. And it is only natural that the increasing insecurities of professional life affect young couples and their approach to parenthood. It is quite common to hear a couple saying that they cannot afford to have a child or any more children. Most couples depend on two incomes to achieve their quality of living yet job security is fast becoming recognized as a thing of the past. The financial burdens associated with having a child are great. All of these pressures and commitments are the reality for today's father-to-be; little wonder that he may well stumble through pregnancy with less enthusiasm and anticipation than he would have liked.

We have a tendency to forget about men when it comes to anything related to pregnancy and childbirth. They, too, need to feel strong and empowered and, just as their partners, to have a support network. The problem is that a man does not receive support from within the existing care system, which is focused mainly on the physical state of the pregnant woman and the baby within. It is my practice to encourage prospective fathers to spend time with me exploring their feelings, hopes and fears – so often completely different to those of mothers-to-be – but, nonetheless, vital to the bigger picture.

All a baby actually needs is to be born into a loving environment, to be kept safe, and to be fed and nurtured. His survival is not contingent on an endless supply of cute clothes, accessories and equipment.

One of the questions I constantly ask myself is how can we shift the huge, impending financial burden from an expectant father's shoulders? Does a young couple really have to live in a spacious house with all the latest mod cons? Could a simpler lifestyle suit a young couple just as well? Maybe these questions are answered by the fact that an increasing number are climbing off the treadmill of an over-demanding career and seeking a simpler option. This often happens after individuals experience a life-changing event such as a birth, when life seems to take on a different perspective.

It is instructive to take a step back and consider the basic requirements of a baby and then compare these to the numerous material expectations we have probably established for ourselves. It is completely possible to provide for a baby's bare necessities without investing large amounts of money; the 50 or so items listed in most pregnancy magazines as the "essentials" are usually nothing of the kind.

If only a father-to-be can be relieved of the pressure of the must-have scenario, I suggest he would then greet the future with eager anticipation. This would be the case in a society that is less demanding financially and more supportive emotionally. To bring about such a situation, employers can play an important role: they can facilitate the forward path by introducing time off work to support a pregnant partner, offer flexi-hours, and provide paid time off when the baby arrives.

The bottom line is that an expectant father, too, needs a supportive network; where there is little or none, he needs to be assured that there's a mechanism to create one. Finding the right balance is imperative if we are ever to hope to manage the increasing level of financial stress associated with parenthood.

Men are naturally protective of their wives or partners and they want what is best for them. But they often make decisions out of ignorance and fear. They don't actually know what the best choices are as this is the first time they have been in this situation. So, apart from the expectant mother wanting to have her issues addressed, the prospective father also needs to have the opportunity to voice his feelings. Feelings are important, and caregivers often tend to focus their attention on the woman at the expense of her partner, who may have very strong feelings that need to be explored. How can a man support his woman if he is feeling frightened or apprehensive? He cannot. The goal should be to ensure fathers are knowledgeable, informed and empowered, and thus able to provide the right backup for their partners.

COMMUNICATING PREGNANCY

For most healthy women, the early signs of pregnancy are one or two missed periods. If you are really in tune with your body, however, you may know even before missing a period. Suddenly, your usual morning cup of coffee or tea tastes "funny", or something deep inside you feels different and you just know.

Until recently, a pregnant woman would share her news early on with her nearest and dearest and they, in turn, would partake of the excitement and anticipation. Other than a varying degree of morning sickness, a lack of periods, and maybe some breast changes, a woman had little else to reassure her that pregnancy was proceeding well – apart from her instinct. She also quietly accepted that her pregnancy could end prematurely or, as in my grandmother's day, that her baby could die at birth or some time in his first year. But, partly due to advances in technology over the last couple of decades, and partly as a result of changing expectations and habits, the way and time at which a woman communicates her pregnancy to her friends and family has changed.

Most women today, suspecting they may be pregnant, use a home pregnancy testing kit to confirm their suspicions. Once pregnancy has been established, the mother-to-be has choices – does she tell everybody about the impending arrival or does she choose, as I believe most nowadays do, to keep the exciting news a secret between her and her partner until her first scan (at around 11 to 13 weeks) reveals a viable pregnancy and a definitive due date? Is this their way of preparing themselves for the disappointment of miscarriage or congenital deformity?

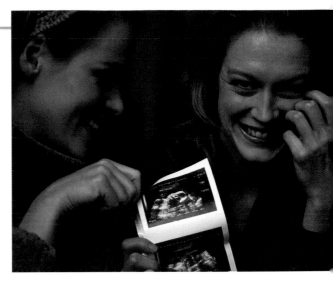

Most of today's pregnant women only share their good news once they have definite "proof" that their babies are alive and well. They probably know this is the case already but are afraid to trust their instincts.

Surely an expectant mother is meant to share the exciting news of a new life with her close family, in order that her emotional needs are sufficiently met and that the safety net of love, comfort and support is available to cushion the fall should anything go wrong? What a shame that this most wonderful and cherished gift is kept a secret for at least its first twelve weeks of existence. Being unable to acknowledge her changed state can affect both the mother-to-be's emotional state – since this is a time a woman can begin the bonding and reassurance process, letting her fetus know how much it is wanted – and also her physical wellbeing. Many pregnant women work, and at the time when they are feeling tired, nauseous, and incapable of delivering their usual level of productivity, they are constrained from sharing the truth with their employers when they most need empathy. Of course, pregnancies do sometimes go wrong and, yes, a higher percentage flounder in the first 12 weeks than at other times, but shouldn't we enter pregnancy with a positive state of mind? And, if something does go wrong, it's really sad that many couples feel they have to deal stoically with their grief in private, instead of reaching out to their network for love and support.

CHANGING RELATIONSHIPS DURING PREGNANCY

Pregnancy and parenthood often bring about significant changes and developments in our perspective towards life, ourselves, and those around us. As a woman prepares to become a mother, a man to become a father, and parents to become grandparents, the dynamics of our personal interactions may evolve quite dramatically. For some women, pregnancy is the ideal opportunity to enhance their wellbeing and spend quality time relaxing and starting to make the mental adjustments that will help to prepare them for motherhood.

Naturally, this is easier for a first pregnancy than for any subsequent one, when the demands of older siblings may restrict the level of quiet, personal time a woman can afford herself.

Pat Thomas's description, see below, is interesting, as it implies once again that our instinctive behaviour, which can naturally provide us with so much strength and guidance during pregnancy, may not be readily accessible due to external factors and the environment in which we live. Most pregnant women, given the chance, will naturally want to do what is best for themselves and for their babies. Basically, if we listen to nature, these needs are very simple. We all need food, shelter and love, but how we achieve them while expecting a baby is very individual. It is indisputable that in order to love and to nurture, we too need to have been loved and nurtured ourselves. While it's nice if that were the case since our own babyhood, some people may not have had that experience. However, I believe it is never too late to start that process, and I'm always very happy to see a new bond struck between expectant parents and their own parents. It is common to hear a woman who has had a baby talk of her new-found appreciation of her mother. Interestingly, this deepening of the child/parent relationship is not exclusive to women. Many men also experience a surge in the bond between them and their parents once a new baby has arrived.

"As a woman your relationship to yourself will have begun to change almost from the moment you knew you were pregnant. It takes a mighty amount of psychological and emotional adjustment to take on board the idea that there is another human life growing inside your body. You may also be more aware of the intuitive side of your nature and your capacity for emotional highs and lows. For the first time your desire to stay true to yourself may clash with the reality of living in a world which encourages conformity."

Alternative Therapy for Pregnancy and Birth by
Pat Thomas

Many women, however, find one of the most challenging aspects of pregnancy arises from having to fend off well-meaning advice from close family! What used to be a natural circle of love, emotional support, and a useful source of information, has become a sticking point for many independent women. This also may be because the average first-time mother is nearer 30 than 20, thus she often does not feel the need to turn to parents who may no longer represent the font of all knowledge in her eyes. Many women are well on the road to total independence by the time they reach thirty, and advice may be well intended but not as welcome as it may have been previously. Also, advice from well-intentioned people will almost always be based on personal experience and hospital practice. As much as this may prove useful, it does not take account of the woman's own instinct.

UNDERSTANDING YOUR PREGNANT STATE

It is funny how much better you understand your parents once you have a child of your own.

Pregnancy is an amazing phenomenon, it involves well-documented physical, emotional and mental changes yet each woman has a unique experience. Pregnancy begins with the union of an egg and sperm, which initiates the production of particular hormones that will allow the pregnancy to be sustained, the baby to grow healthily within his mother, and the body to start preparing itself for birth and motherhood. The way a woman reacts to pregnancy and its associated changes will be different from woman to woman, just as it can be different from pregnancy to pregnancy in the same woman. However, many women think that a differing pregnancy can signal a child of the opposite sex.

I am unaware of any research into hormonal and/or chemical balance or imbalance that is created by, or influenced by, the sex of an unborn baby. Nor do the changes in a woman's shape as pregnancy advances or whether she carries more to the front or to the side indicate her baby's sex. Increasingly, however, I hear women say that instinctively they know the sex of their babies. While I have observed over the years that many mothers who suffer greatly with morning sickness with a baby of one sex have hardly been affected when carrying a baby of the opposite sex, this is not a deciding indicator, as some women endure the same, sometimes extreme pregnancy side effects, no

I recall when I was expecting my last baby; everything about the pregnancy seemed to be different compared to the others. Mostly it was that the degree of morning – or should I say, all day – sickness was markedly less. As my baby grew inside me, many people remarked that my shape was different. So, in the still of the night, I secretly began to think that with three fine sons already, maybe this one just might be a girl. Not, I hasten to add, were we "trying" for a girl. My instincts did not support my fantasies and rightly so, for my fourth baby was another beautiful son!

> **There is an overwhelming advantage for a newly pregnant woman to be able to discuss with a knowledgeable health professional her early pregnancy symptoms and the possible ways and means they could be minimized.**

matter what the sex of the baby. I believe as a woman increases her family so, too, grows her wisdom, knowledge and awareness of the miracle of pregnancy and birth. This awareness, combined with the accompanying physical, psychological and emotional changes, results in each pregnancy being unique, as no two are ever the same.

SYMPTOMS OF PREGNANCY

Some of the common physical effects that women often notice when pregnant, especially in early pregnancy, are overwhelming tiredness, breast changes (which often become more sensitive as they would before menstruation); changes in stools; nausea or sickness and also a changing taste in the mouth.

From an emotional perspective, you may be feeling a little pre-menstrual, in the same way you may before a period. Hormonal changes can result in more obvious sways of emotion. This does not apply to all women but is not to be a cause of concern if it does! It is all quite normal and is just nature's way of preparing you and your body for the next few months. It is interesting how many people complain about being pregnant for nine months; when you actually think about everything the mind and the body have to prepare for, it is a miracle we can do it in such a short space of time!

That being said, however, I still believe it unfortunate that many of today's mothers-to-be wish to conceal their pregnancies until after their first scans and sometimes, even after their second! This is because, from early on, there often are a number of side effects that can and should be looked after. Chief among them is

Some years ago, I was midwife to Caroline who, from the earliest weeks of her first pregnancy, suffered from excessive salivation to the extent that she spent her waking hours with a container in one hand for the saliva and a filled water bottle in the other. This extreme symptom disappeared immediately after the birth of her healthy baby. Her second pregnancy progressed without such debilitation even though she had the same-sex baby.

There are a large number of hormones that have specific functions in pregnancy. Some are present in the body all the time, others are released during pregnancy. Many of the side effects of pregnancy are a result of their actions.

HCG (*human chorionic gonadotrophin*) is widely known as the "pregnancy hormone", because it is the one that is tested for in pregnancy tests. It is released by the developing placenta as it begins to implant within the uterus. It triggers other hormonal activity needed to maintain your pregnancy and prevents menstruation from occurring.

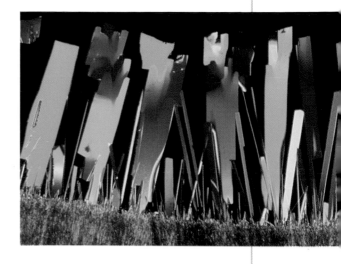

Progesterone plays an important role in sustaining your pregnancy, including preventing the uterus from contracting strongly. At around 8 to 9 weeks of pregnancy, the placenta begins to produce it in large quantities.

Oestrogen helps to prepare the lining of the uterus for the pregnancy, increasing the number of blood vessels and glands present within the uterus.

tiredness. If an expectant mother does not rest or sleep at every available opportunity, she will not only be overwhelmed by fatigue but it will exacerbate all her other possible minor disorders.

Usually, you will find that by 14-16 weeks of pregnancy, the majority of the early symptoms have started to diminish, if they have not disappeared altogether. At this stage, you will often find that you enter a more energetic phase, feeling more like you did prior to being pregnant. But, as every woman is different, what symptoms she has, and the times they'll occur and subside will vary. Not only will symptoms vary from woman to woman but also from pregnancy to pregnancy. The important fact to remember is that all these feelings are normal and individual. Your partner may tease and claim he does not recognize the woman who now greets him each night, but rest assured we have all been there! Inconsistent behaviour, memory loss, persistent scattiness, and inexplicable ups and downs are typical complaints from many pregnant woman (and their partners). Look at it in the same positive way you look at your growing tummy – a sign that all is well as your mind and body concentrate on the development of the baby inside you.

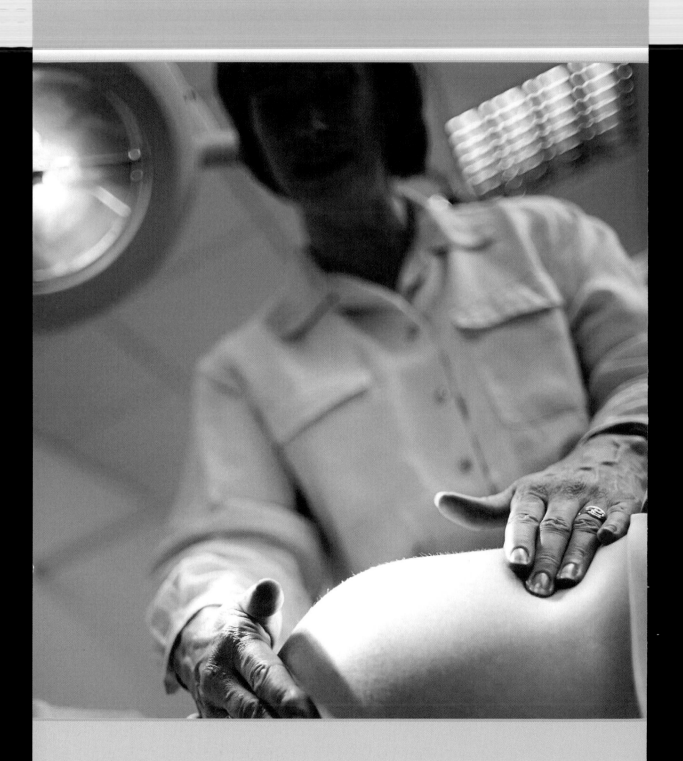

CHAPTER 2
Informed Choice

Whenever I talk about "the system", I am referring to the standard or routine care available to pregnant women. Although there are differences in each country's provision of care and what comes as "standard" – childbirth not being covered by private medical insurance in the UK unless a specific operative procedure becomes necessary while maternity care is provided as part of the medical insurance that is paid for by each individual in the USA and Switzerland – generally, the tendency has been to medicalize childbirth and for routine care to centre around procedures that favour practitioner and hospital practice rather than the needs of individual expectant mothers.

CHANGES IN CHILDBIRTH

Over the years, many events have impacted on the health and welfare of pregnant mothers and their babies. Among the most significant was the realization during the 19th century that infection could be controlled. Prior to this time, childbirth was extremely hazardous, with thousands of mothers perishing from puerperal fever. Sadly, early-day midwives did not have the benefit of appropriate research and technology to complement their basic skills, nor were there sufficient antenatal and postnatal care support services.

Another transforming policy was the introduction in England in 1902 of formal training programmes for midwives, replacing lay midwives, which acknowledged the importance of good antenatal care, coupled with innovative medical discoveries, such as blood transfusions and antibiotics. All these contributed to the improvement in the safety and benefits of maternity care for women. These were very important discoveries at the time, and greatly improved the outcome for many mothers and their babies.

Trained midwives were thus able to care for pregnant women in a more knowledgeable way, accumulating skills, experience, and strengthened instincts as they progressed through their careers. The

EARLY BIRTH

Midwife comes from the Anglo-Saxon "mid-wif" meaning with women. It is an ancient profession, as childbirth was naturally the provenance of women. In ancient Greece, in order to be a midwife you had to have given birth yourself, though until the early 20th century, there was no other legal requirement to assist at birth. The first mention of a midwife in English history is in the 12th-century chronicle, Historia Anglorum, which refers to an ancient Briton woman placing girdles, imbued with supernatural powers, about the bellies of women during difficult labours. Men gradually began to assume a role in childbirth, and by the Victorian era, most middle- and upper-class woman had switched to being attended by doctors, all of whom were male. Louis XIII of France's wish to view the process is reputed to be behind the quiet acceptance of European women to lay on their backs to deliver their babies.

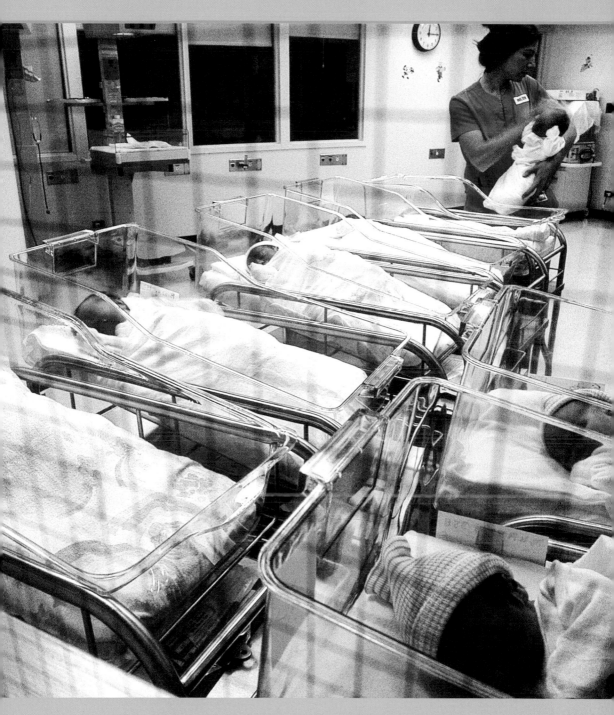

Massed ranks of babies are more an image of an earlier age when childbirth was more regimented than it can be today — provided the right choices are made.

local district midwife became a well-known figure to families in her surrounding neighbourhood. She was respected as a truly hands-on professional – expert in normal pregnancy and childbirth. Between the 1900s and early 1970s, midwives were encouraged to use their unique accumulated skills and developing instincts. This, coupled with a sound training programme, provided increased benefit to all mothers in their care. A midwife was regarded not only as a birth educator and deliverer of babies, but also as a breastfeeding expert, marriage counsellor and confidante. Home birth rates were high; once women had successfully delivered their first babies in the hospital, they were encouraged to deliver subsequent babies at home.

Between 1900 and the early 1970s, birth was not medicalized. Not only were hospital beds lacking but scanning machines and monitors had yet to be invented. This was the heyday of the district midwife, who was known, trusted and respected. Mothers saw her as a familiar face and the midwife, in spite of long hours, had infinite job satisfaction and was a respected pillar of the community. I often ask myself whether these years when the district midwife travelled around on her bicycle delivering babies at home were "the good days" or were we living in naïve ignorance of potential dangers yet unknown? Mothers then accepted they could, or their baby could, die during the process of childbirth, and even two generations ago, this remained an accepted risk. Many women, especially in the absence of contraception, expected to continue having babies throughout their fertile years, and possibly lose one or two as a matter of course.

However, beginning in the 1970s in the UK, and earlier in the US, political opinion began to advocate hospital births, as they were seen as the safest option. Hospitals and obstetricians were encouraged to aim for 100 per cent hospital births. Mothers who wanted to continue having babies at their home found it increasingly difficult to do so as the years went by, not least because community midwives were losing their confidence in supporting women. They began encouraging mothers to adhere to the new policies. This process resulted in a plummeting level in home births and a resultant loss of skills by midwives. During these decades, only a few midwives were still able to offer mothers informed choice.

Interestingly, in 1993 the Royal College of Gynaecologists published a paper stating that home birth is a safe option and, in some instances, safer than hospitals. This finding was substantiated through further research by the National Birthday Trust (1997), which concluded that the perinatal mortality rate for hospital births was higher than for home births.

The midwives that train now, unless they are of an exceptional calibre, only feel confident with technology in close proximity. Today's student midwives are educated primarily in universities, the emphasis seemingly being on the theoretical aspects of pregnancy and childbirth, and there is only a fraction of the "hands on" practical

* Before I was a mother or midwife, I was staying with my sister, Jennifer, who was expecting her second baby. Just before dawn, my brother-in-law awakened me with the news that Jen was in labour. He set off with undue haste to milk his cows having summoned the district midwife. Soon, a seemingly elderly lady with her sleeves rolled up appeared and sent me off to boil a kettle of water – to this day, I don't know for what purpose! As a result, I missed the somewhat swift birth of my second nephew. Following the birth, Jennifer was tucked up in her own bed with my nephew happily nursing at her breast. I don't imagine for one minute that she, like other midwives of the time, carried all the resuscitation equipment that today's midwives do and, had something gone wrong, she would have been of limited help. Having said that, I have no doubt that this wise, experienced midwife safely managed many an unforeseen circumstance, such as an undiagnosed breech birth.

midwifery training of yesteryear. While today's students graduate with increased technological skills, they soon become aware that there is less opportunity to be with women, and this has a demoralizing effect, which may be why there is a dramatic shortage of midwives.

THE ROLE OF THE FAMILY DOCTOR

Previously, your local GP (general practitioner) also had an all-important part to play, alongside the midwife, as it was he who continued to care for a woman long after the midwife had left. GPs played a pivotal role in caring for their patients when they became pregnant, with many enjoying the obstetrical side. They were fulfilled by the fact that they attended the birth of another generation of their practice. Your mother, and certainly your grandmother, may be able to tell you of the family's doctor, and how he looked after the family's medical problems and may even have been present at your birth. He knew the family and, more importantly, the family history. How satisfying that was for patient and doctor. Familiarity and trust, strengthened by a mother's instinct about her family, produced medical care that took more account of the individual. Furthermore, respect between the professions was very high; midwives and GPs often worked in tandem, complementing and learning from each other. Continuity of care for the pregnant woman was assured by the trusted district community midwife, who was closely supported during pregnancy and often the birth itself by the GP. Change in the political climate and the way in which GPs now practice has made this continuum of care virtually impossible to sustain. These days, GPs are almost always part of an ever-growing consortium, providing fragmented and often faceless care. The time available to patients by even the most dedicated GP is limited, and GPs are becoming increasingly distanced from "their" patients. The present fragmentation of care often results in an individual being unable to see her own GP at a time when she needs to consult a professional who possesses a knowledge of both her medical history and personal background.

Another explanation for the erosion of GP maternity care is the training now provided to doctors and the beliefs that are inherently imparted. GPs have become reluctant to offer pregnant women the complete and transparent portfolio of informed choice, because they fear that should a woman elect to birth her baby at home and there is some deviation from normal during the labour or birth, they may be held accountable for the outcome. This is actually not the case, yet it is easy to understand the natural fear of a GP, given the bias of his or her training based on a medical approach governed by modern-day obstetrics, rather than through knowledge and experience acquired from observing and participating in natural and normal childbirth. If a GP is requested to attend a home birth by the midwife he cannot refuse but, generally, midwives now accept the limited obstetric experience of most GPs and would not recommend nor request their attendance. In fact, midwives feel more confident in the knowledge that should a home birth deviate from normal, it is safer to transfer to the hospital in an equipped ambulance attended by trained paramedics.

When I was a community midwife, I hastily established contact with any new GP in the hope that he or she may have been interested in mother-centred care and the possibility of home birth as a safe option. Those who showed an interest soon voluntarily became involved in providing GP backup to the mothers in their practices who had decided to have a home birth. I only requested their attendance when the mother was approaching or in the second stage of her labour. As a consequence, I was able to share many magical moments with these GPs, who all commented how fulfilling and inspirational their experiences were. Two GPs in particular paid me the compliment of asking me to attend the births of their wives when they decided on home birth. One of them is my own GP. Opposite, you can read what he has to say.

The sad reality is that most GPs are not actively encouraged in this way and the fulfilment described above is rare to come by. The medical system imposed today dictates the activities of the various health professionals. The majority of us in the profession believe our roles have become less rewarding. Our basic desire to care is in conflict with the requirements of conforming to bureaucratic administration.

When I entered general practice, my experience of obstetrics was limited to the short and distorted education offered at medical school, along with six months' exposure as a junior hospital doctor arranging and supporting augmented labours and instrumental deliveries. Imagine my bewilderment and shock as a new GP, to discover women asking to have their babies at home.

I was fortunate to be taken in hand by Val, working as a midwife attached to our practice, whose philosophy matched my own aims of patient-centred and holistic care. I was able to make time to work alongside Val to experience the management of home confinements. What I discovered was not hospital midwifery taken into the community, but a higher level of practitioner-patient communication; peaceful and naturally-paced deliveries by mothers acting with confidence, and enhanced by their home surroundings.

There was little for me to do, other than observe and learn as the midwife and mother worked so closely. Observation allowed more insights into natural childbirth than the last-minute rush of medical student deliveries, and the instrumental deliveries of the junior doctor allowed. I thought "transition" was only to be found in textbooks and certainly not in the noise and anxiety of the labour ward until I witnessed natural home confinement. Here, less fearful mothers progressed through labour's finely tuned stages in familiar surroundings.

For many, both professionals and women, there are great fears regarding the safety of home confinements. The clear imbalance in the perception of risk and the outcome measure is reassuring to me. Far greater than statistics is that responsibility for selection, preparation, monitoring, and decision-making is shared by a competent and skilled midwife and an informed mother. That responsibility is focussed to a greater level of detail and performance than is often seen with "normal" deliveries in hospital obstetric units. If problems arise, and they do, a full range of equipment and transfer arrangements are available in the home. What is the role of the family doctor in the future of community obstetrics? Diagnosis is our natural field, but it could include pre-conceptual counselling, shared antenatal care, a role in the delivery for those GPs with a special interest, shared postnatal care, and baby checks. The outcome of working with a mother and family during this natural life experience adds colour and depth to the doctor-patient relationship, which can be retained for a lifetime.

THE POLITICS OF CHILDBIRTH

Politics has had a direct influence on how the medical profession treats maternal care and consequently where women birth their babies. In the UK and the USA, the surge in hospital births in the latter half of the 20th century was perpetuated by information disseminated to women by the government and medical practitioners. Many of the new ideas and approaches toward birth were introduced from America. There, medical insurance and private funding were directed at obstetric care and, as a result, many of the new tools and techniques used in the United States were exported to Europe. Along with these advances, however, also came some less positive factors. Increasing use of litigation put significant pressure on any organization working within the public domain and none more so than those responsible for bringing new babies into the world. A fear of litigation and huge damage claims soon began to force hospitals to formulate and engage in practices that they could deem "safe". Restrictive policies and procedures started to be imposed on all women, often at the expense of allowing them the freedom to follow their natural instincts.

There was also much good in what research into and development of Western obstetrics could provide. Many things that were inconceivable 20 years ago are almost commonplace today, such as babies being born at 24 weeks having an unprecedented chance of survival, and operations performed in utero or immediately after birth to correct physical abnormalities discovered during routine scans. Neonatal care has made such significant advances that more and more young lives are being saved all the time. It is truly amazing what we have learnt to do with knowledge and technology and such progress is to be acclaimed.

In our age of more open and accessible communication, communities of scientists now work across geographic boundaries. The result is that obstetric experts now interact in a way that creates pools of knowledge, bringing together all the individual pockets of research and expertise to develop a universal knowledge base that encompasses a wide spectrum of information. This is technology used at its best, opening channels of communication and providing universal access to information. Modern-day obstetrics is heavily dependent on technology and, while this has created many of the miracles for which we are so grateful, it also has led to the erosion of some of the instinctive behaviour and basic knowledge that made childbirth the amazing event that nature intended.

As recently as the summer of 2004, a highly skilled midwife was dismissed by the hospital that employed him for supporting a mother having a home birth.

USE OF TECHNOLOGY

When we refer to technology in pregnancy we are really referring to the use of monitors and scans, as well as blood testing. We also may think of technological intervention, such as epidurals, caesarean sections, and drug-based labour inductions, but these will be discussed later in chapter 7.

The use of monitors demonstrates how quickly and pervasively technology can influence the course of childbirth. The UK first began importing monitors from the USA in the early 1970s, although at the time we were assured that their use would be limited to high-risk mothers only. Over the decades, monitors became central to all expectant mothers' care; the larger hospitals installed major terminals, which display information received from individual monitors beside each woman's bed. These central observation terminals can be observed by midwives and doctors, and they reduce the need for bedside care. The inevitable result is that women become more and more isolated, and the midwife less skilled.

However, it has recently been stated that a skilled, experienced midwife can, in some instances, be better than a CTG (cardiotocograph) machine. Machines are fallible and only truly accurate if interpreted by an expert practitioner who is present throughout its use. Wrong interpretation can result in either appropriate intervention coming too late or many unnecessary caesarean sections. How often have I heard fathers say that they were requested to observe the monitor and call for help if they were worried!

We have almost arrived back at square one with monitors. While they definitely have their place for monitoring high-risk situations, they should not be used as a routine check on the natural progression of a woman in healthy labour. The greater use of epidurals, however, may be responsible for their continued widespread use. The only way of ascertaining whether a woman under epidural anaesthetic is having a contraction, is to see the reaction on the monitor. The one is perpetuating the other.

That being said, I'm all in favour of the appropriate use of technology; without it many pregnancies would result in a catastrophic outcome for mother or baby, or even both. However, it is important to take note of the word "appropriate", and this may be even more apposite when I discuss the use of ultrasonography or scanning.

SCANNING

Ultrasonography involves bouncing high-frequency sound waves off soft matter. In pregnancy, such soft matter is your baby. In the UK, "routine" scans are performed twice during a normal singleton pregnancy. At time of writing this book, the first is performed between 11 and 13 weeks when the growing baby can be seen on screen. In most hospitals now, this first scan is called the "nuchal" scan. During the scan, the sonographer will pinpoint a certain area at the back of your baby's neck, known as the nuchal fold. A picture of this area will be taken and measurements of the area done and plotted against the age of the mother in order to establish a percentage chance of your baby having the chromosomal abnormality, Down syndrome. Research has proved this an early indicator.

When a woman is being monitored using the CTG machine, she is denied the freedom to move further than the leads will allow and the focus of attention shifts from her to the machine.

Although a nuchal scan will not provide a definitive answer, by being given a ball-park percentage, you may have grounds upon which to decide to proceed with more invasive procedures, such as CVS (Chorionic Villus Sampling) or Amniocentesis.

A nuchal scan measurement gives you a statistic, your risk factor or one-in-something chance of producing a child with Down syndrome. If you fall into the high-risk band, you are faced with the dilemma of "What do we do now? Do we accept the fact that this baby could be a Down's baby?" Or do you submit yourself to a more definitive diagnostic procedure such as CVS or amniocentesis, invasive procedures associated with a miscarriage rate dependent on the obstetrician and his skill?

In the UK, the 20-week scan, as it used to be called, is now being performed later – up to 23 weeks, and is more commonly termed the "anomaly scan". Again, it is designed to reaffirm the normality of the baby and the pregnancy. The baby is measured from every conceivable angle and the results documented. The placenta's position also

DIAGNOSTIC TESTS

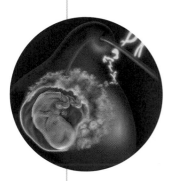

CVS can be performed as early as 11 to 13 weeks into the pregnancy to detect genetic and chromosomal abnormalities. A small piece of the placenta is removed through a fine needle inserted either through the cervix or, under local anaesthetic, into the abdomen. The risk of miscarriage associated with this procedure is about one percent.

Amniocentesis can detect neural tube disorders in addition to genetic problems. It is usually performed from 16 weeks onwards. A fine needle is used to extract a small quantity of amniotic fluid through the abdomen. The cells in the fluid are cultured in a laboratory over a few days and checked for abnormal chromosomes. It has a slightly lower risk of miscarriage than CVS.

will be identified. It is reassuring for both caregiver and expectant mother to know that it is not in a potentially hazardous position.

I believe that the womb is a sanctuary, and that it should not be entered into without valid reason. Couples should be counselled and approval sought before any procedure – even those considered noninvasive – is undertaken. Every couple, however, will have a different definition of "valid". Most believe that detecting an anomaly in utero could result in a lifesaving decision, and this may be deemed a valid reason for undergoing a scan. The nuchal scan tends to be a little more contentious as this determines the accuracy of dates and provides a risk assessment. But if a couple are certain they would welcome their baby irrespective of whether or not he has a chromosomal abnormality, this scan would be of little importance. Of course, in this day and age couples want and expect a perfect baby, so the nuchal scan becomes of great relevance.

The amazing abilities of today's sophisticated scanning equipment are to be marvelled at. Detection of abnormality is becoming increasingly accurate. The question of safety, however, is often raised. We know that scanning is safer than X-rays and, to date, there has been no definitive proof that babies suffer physically from this procedure. Research continues, however, as concern has been expressed regarding the impact heavy scanning could have on a baby's hearing, but again this has not been proven. Scanning is a technological tool that can provide essential information and even save lives, yet it should not be used without the couple understanding the purpose of the procedure. A couple expecting a baby will be very vulnerable to any information they are given, yet it is not uncommon for scans to be read incorrectly. And what exactly do statistics mean in

A young couple once re-booked with our practice. Already the parents of a lively two year old, they didn't really want to know the sex of their unborn baby, but it was unexpectedly revealed by the sonographer that it was 99.9 percent certain they were expecting a girl. At the birth, I heard the father gasp "It's a boy!" in disbelief. This little baby was welcomed into the family but the parents still grieved for the daughter they no longer had, and for many weeks the older brother invited visitors to see his baby sister.

pregnancy? It does not matter how much outcomes can be improved, some people always have to form the majority, and some people the minority.

BLOOD TESTING

This is another area that falls under the umbrella of technology; early blood tests are routinely carried out for every expectant mother unless she refuses. The question of blood testing is increasingly complex and, in some instances, slightly controversial (such as HIV testing). Blood testing is of obvious value because it determines the mother's blood group (if she doesn't already know it), and more importantly, her rhesus factor, and the possibility of anaemia. Because of the way we can now break down and investigate blood, it is possible to find out if a woman's blood cells are the right shape, size and quantity, have sufficient red and white cells, and ascertain their exact composition in order to ensure a healthy pregnancy and baby.

Although there is no risk of harm to a woman or her baby in having blood tests and, moreover, while they provide important information that is particularly useful in emergencies, I still think that a woman should consent to blood tests through informed decision making. She needs to be aware of the reasons and advantages that support these tests; too often, these procedures are undertaken without question, all in the name of routine. If we involve an expectant mother in the decision-making process right from the start, she will feel respected and involved.

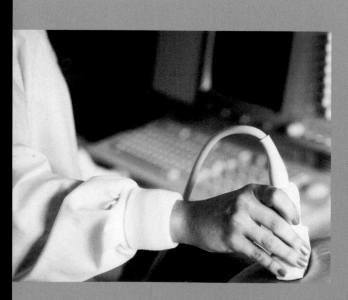

It's always a thrill to see your baby, particularly if he is moving around. We now know that babies as young as 9 to 11 weeks of gestation are capable of sophisticated movements such as kicking, stepping and jumping. Ultrasound scans can help parents bond with their unborn babies and certainly help to alleviate parents' fears.

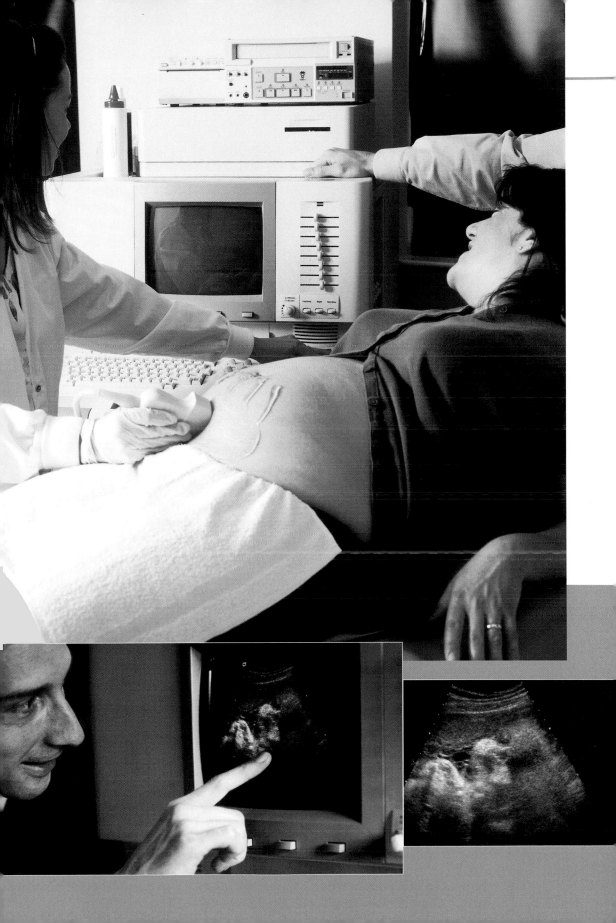

THE HUMAN FACTOR

In many ways, we have seen the focus of investment shifting away from human care, such as midwives, in favour of technology. We have accelerated the potential demise of more instinctive midwives – who approach birthing as a natural experience that needs support but little interference from them – by encouraging midwives to undertake tasks previously performed by doctors. Examples include suturing, siting intravenous drips and scanning. While this is innovative practice for some midwives and, in many ways, a midwife is the best person to administer these procedures, I believe the decision to perform such tasks should really be left to each individual midwife. Many midwives would see these procedures as digressing from the core skills associated with the true art of midwifery, and thus would see this as a route they would not wish to follow.

The majority of midwives enter the profession with the overwhelming desire to be with women; after all, that is the definition of a midwife! They want to develop midwifery skills by creating a trusting relationship with "their" women that can largely only be achieved with one-to-one midwifery. To develop these skills – to listen to the unborn baby's heartbeat and detect when it is abnormal, to place a hand on a labouring mother's abdomen and be able to divine the frequency and intensity of the contractions, to listen and understand a woman's needs and safely guide and support her through a technology-free pregnancy, labour and birth – the midwife needs time, a very rare commodity these days.

Think about using technology to your advantage as a tool to support your own instinct as opposed to relying on it to tell you everything you need to know about your baby.

In fairness to obstetricians, there are some who are totally supportive of midwives retrieving their unique role of expert practitioners of normal pregnancy providing total care for pregnant mothers, and requesting obstetric opinion only when concern or deviation from the norm arises. However, midwives themselves are sometimes reluctant to accept this responsibility and, to a certain extent, reliance on technological innovations has resulted in otherwise confident and competent midwives having their core skills eroded.

My biggest lament over the use of technology is that it is now used routinely with little or no explanation of its advantages and disadvantages. My message is clear: not all technology is appropriate although many mothers and their babies can directly praise its use for a safe outcome and a miracle that may not otherwise have happened.

✳   Erin was 26 weeks pregnant when she contacted me to say that she was concerned but unsure as to why. Erin had the routine scans at 11 and 23 weeks, which confirmed a normal, apparently healthy, pregnancy. Erin already had a two-year-old son, born by emergency caesarean section, and she was keen to experience a vaginal birth this time.

My examination revealed no apparent problems but abdominal palpation indicated a slight excess of liquor (the fluid surrounding the baby). The family were about to go on a much-needed holiday, so we agreed that I would make an appointment for Erin to have a scan on her return. This scan revealed a dramatic increase in the liquor volume, which had largely occurred in the preceding week. She was swiftly transferred to the hospital where the excess fluid was successfully drained.

Unfortunately, this was only the beginning of a progressive complication of Erin's pregnancy due to a rare placental growth. She was, however, subsequently successfully delivered of a daughter at term.

Her baby appeared healthy at birth but became increasingly jaundiced over the next months. No cause could be found and no treatment could be offered. Erin wanted her baby at home and kept insisting "My baby will get better" – even though I thought otherwise. However, get well she did. Breast milk and a mother's love resulted in the jaundice receding gradually over the following five months. By her first birthday, she was a happy, healthy baby.

ENTERING "THE SYSTEM"

Is it possible for any first-time mother-to-be to fully understand the prevailing ante- and postnatal system, one that is quite complex in nature and upon which the majority of us are totally dependent? Although most maternity units claim to support every mother with a philosophy of care that allows her to be involved in decision making, the wording of most of these pledges is very ambiguous and the reality far from the intent. Inevitably, the mother-to-be in the early stages of pregnancy, finds herself bewildered by her encounters with an impersonal bureaucracy, as the majority of present-day maternity units are no longer small, intimate birthing units of previous times, but large hospital departments whose culture is far from one of caring intimacy. Imagine a scenario where your doctor says: "There are many options available to you for the birth of your baby. For the birth of their first babies many women opt to go into the hospital, but if you are assertive and interested, there are other alternatives. In this area we are very lucky to have a midwifery-led unit, a private birthing centre, and a group of independent midwives with an excellent reputation. This means you could have your baby in the hospital, in a specialized birthing unit, or even at home. What I can do is provide you with all the relevant information and contact details, in order that you can take the time to think about it over the next few months and discuss with your partner where you feel the most appropriate place would be." In other words, your doctor takes the responsibility for outlining all the available options in the area, be they private or state-funded. Although it is unlikely you are ready to make a decision there and then, at least you leave the surgery understanding what your options are and how you can contact the relevant individuals.

A nice scenario, but quite different from the reality of what most mothers-to-be will experience during the first three months of pregnancy.

CONSULTING YOUR GP

In the UK, a woman's first port of call is her GP's surgery, which, as a practicing body, has slowly become more and more fragmented. One of the frustrating factors that has resulted from the fragmentation of GP practices is that when a woman first finds out she is pregnant and books to see her GP, her doctor may not be familiar with his or her patient. As a result, a woman could well be going to see a strange GP to announce her pregnancy and receive the first stage of her prenatal care. Is the GP going to know whether or not the couple has had a long period of infertility, and thus be able to be congratulatory and supporting? Is he or she going to know whether this mother is in a stable relationship, or if she is not in a relationship at all, in which case she may not consider this pregnancy good news? How does a GP know how to respond if this is their first meeting, and how much time can the doctor afford whatever the scenario?

Generally, a pregnant woman will be given the standard ten-minute slot to sit and tell her GP that she is pregnant and offload all her initial questions about this huge change that is taking place inside her and the subsequent events. If she is lucky, she will have a comprehensive list of enquiries that she ticks off as her doctor provides her with the information she requires. (Very few GPs have heard of independent midwives.) If she is unlucky, her GP will give her a copy of standard literature and tell her that all the answers to her questions can be found within and will be answered by the hospital at her booking-in visit, somewhere between 11 and 15 weeks.

The main talking point during this first session will be the name of the hospital to which the mother would like to be referred. Having discussed this, the doctor says: "I

Heidi, aged 37, was excitedly pregnant for the first time, having been told that it would be highly unlikely she would ever have children. She was 30 weeks into her pregnancy when we first met for a consultation. Her story was one of utter frustration. Her medical history, on face value, appeared daunting. In the past, she had successful brain surgery for a benign tumour, which sadly left her suffering with severe epilepsy. Further surgery cured the frequent seizures and she'd not had one for ten years. However, she did suffer from severe depression, for which she was treated with strong medication to control her mood swings.

Once pregnant, Heidi decided, without medical advice, to stop all medication. Instinctively believing that as a miracle pregnancy had happened, she could now progress on her own – and she did. Remarkably, her much wanted pregnancy advanced without complication except for an increasingly debilitating condition called symphysis pubis dysfunction, which interfered with normal walking so she had to use crutches.

Heidi was definitely high risk but she dreamed of a home water birth and her instincts were telling her it was a safe option. I listened intently; she was passionate about trusting her instincts. I advised Heidi that my philosophy of care is "healthy mother, healthy baby, and a safe birth", even if it means intervention, but that the intervention would be appropriate and timely, and she would be involved in the decision-making. She understood and agreed and I then consented to be her midwife.

At term plus three days, with the pool in place, Heidi called me to attend her. Contractions were now fairly frequent. She laboured in the pool by candlelight, with her husband's arms wrapped safely around her. The hours slipped by; mother and baby were fine but progress was very slow. Heidi found it increasingly difficult to cope with the strong contractions. We assessed the situation and Heidi decided to transfer to the hospital and to have an epidural. Although pain-free, her progress remained very slow, and her baby's heart rate was beginning to signal distress. Heidi agreed with the decision that a caesarean section would be the safest way for her baby to be born. Three days later she returned home with a beautiful 9-lb son. When three days after her long labour I asked her how she felt emotionally, she replied "Deeply fulfilled".

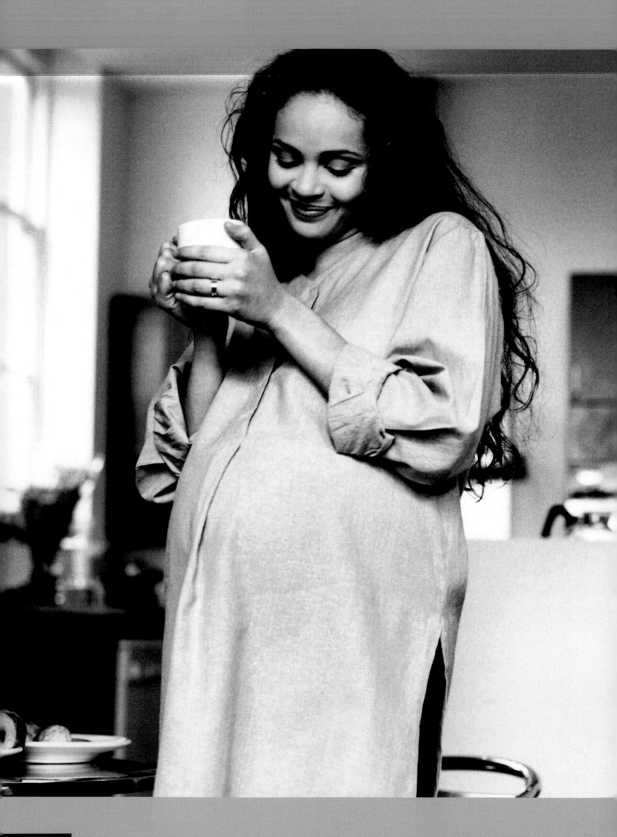

will write a referral letter for you and you will receive an appointment from the hospital." The mother may then wait six weeks before she has the opportunity to talk to anyone else in the "profession" about her pregnancy. With whom, therefore, can she sit down and talk through the complexities of scans and blood tests, their advantages and disadvantages, without bias? How can the mother-to-be equip herself with the necessary knowledge and information that places her in a strong position to be involved in decision-making about her and her baby? If she has the opportunity to explore the options, she is far less likely to be carried along with the routine of pregnancy monitoring, and more likely to feel that she has a strong voice to be heard and for her instincts to be aroused.

THE NON-CONTINUITY OF CARE

At this amazing stage in her life, a woman's instincts start to emerge and an ever-increasing number of questions start to materialize. To whom does she turn? In the first few months, unless she has opted for private obstetric care, it is unlikely she has been provided with a dedicated contact that she can call and with whom she can discuss any questions or concerns. And what about the mother-to-be who may not have been properly advised? Once a woman has gone through the process of booking herself in, either within the state- or the privately-controlled sector, she will then be subject to the appointment schedule, scanning procedures, and tests of that particular system.

It would appear that most obstetricians, who are experts of the abnormal, have their own ideas as to when routine procedures should be performed and how often the mother-to-be needs to be seen and by whom. For once a mother has booked for private care with an obstetrician, her appointments will often be brief, devoid of choice, and as frequent as the physician feels appropriate.

In the UK, faced with hospital cutbacks and the apparent disarray in the health service, pregnant mothers are often not seen early enough in their pregnancies, a crucial time when health education can be offered and, more importantly, feelings explored. This is, I believe, the time when the mother should meet the community-based caring midwife, who will support the mother throughout her pregnancy. In certain areas in the UK, the booking-in time is changing from 12 weeks to 8 weeks. This is great news for mothers, as they will be able to share some of their questions, thoughts and concerns with an understanding midwife who is going to be very supportive about their pregnancies. Moreover, if anything untoward should happen, these women are going to have midwives with whom they can share their loss and distress.

The apparent universally accepted pattern of antenatal care, unless there is a medical or obstetric deviation, is that the mother-to-be is seen approximately three to four times until 28 weeks. Then more regularly until 36 weeks, after which she is seen weekly. The question I have is whether this pattern is sufficient to embrace the care and attention that is every woman's right. Generally, the level of contact with a practitioner is very low and you may or may not see the same person more than once. The result is that throughout pregnancy there is no one to listen to your questions, no one to ask how you are feeling, no one to encourage you to begin to trust your own body and instincts.

In my experience the last ten weeks of pregnancy is the most crucial time for the mother-to-be. This is when the partnership between her and her midwife should strengthen as they start to focus on the weeks ahead. This relationship should be conducted at a pace dictated only by the mother and her instinct, as she prepares herself for the most important day of her life – her baby's birth. However, the reality in these days of financial constraints and shortage of midwives, is that often there is no partnership of care. But if you are lucky enough to find a midwife who will support you, the positive impact this will have on these last few weeks, will influence your approach to labour and birth forever.

Finding a midwife in the system who will become your partner and help you to fulfil your birthing aspirations is a lottery which you may or may not win.

Yet in our perceived bid to make progress for the good of mothers and babies, I feel we have ignored the most important factor of all. That is the woman's instinct and her intuitive ability to make an informed choice once all the options are presented in a factual and unbiased manner. When I think of a mother who is about to enter "the system" during her first pregnancy, I wonder how or if she could know whether the doctor's referral to the hospital is the right choice for her? So, uninformed and ill-advised, she enters "the system".

"The system" itself tends to be pretty pre-determined, and the natural feeling is one of joining a conveyor belt. Although it may be your first pregnancy and quite possibly the most important and exciting event of your life, this is "business as usual" for the establishment you are in. There is very little time for the woman to be put at ease by a qualified midwife, whom she will gradually get to know and trust. In a similar vein, there is little time these days in which a midwife can use her own skills and instinct to encourage knowledge and understanding in the woman in her care in order for the midwife to successfully "monitor" her patient's progress and foresee any potential problem. This is not a criticism directed at midwives but at the current system, as I am sure that, given the chance, most midwives would probably like to be the named midwife for a number of women in their care.

Suzi enjoyed her first pregnancy, which was straightforward and uncomplicated, and was delighted when her labour began soon after her due date. She called the local maternity unit at what she perceived to be a timely moment, and was advised to go in, which she did. Eight hours later she was delivered of a lovely baby girl and was discharged two days later. On her return home, however, she gradually developed severe postnatal depression, which not only affected her ability to mother her baby, but also put a great strain on her marriage. Her depressive illness lasted two years.

I became her midwife when she was newly pregnant with her second baby four years later. I reviewed her previous birth experience with her moment by moment. It became apparent to me that although Suzi's labour was straightforward, an almost textbook experience to a midwife, for Suzi it had been a nightmare of conforming to the midwife's wishes. She had attempted many times in her labour to vocalize her wishes to be mobile – to stand, kneel, or squat, but it hadn't happened, and this normally assertive woman's instinctive voice was silenced with quite dramatic lasting effects.

Suzi was now afraid that the post-natal depression would return, and she did not want to go into the hospital. Working one-to-one, however, we gradually formed a trusting partnership. This was particularly fortunate as her husband was exceedingly reluctant to be involved in the pregnancy, labour or birth – Suzi's previous experience had taken its toll on him.

Suzi's second baby, a boy, was born safely at home at 42 weeks, weighing 10 lbs 4 oz – and yes, her husband and daughter were there for the birth. She had no evidence of depression. Some weeks later we talked through the birth notes giving Suzi every opportunity to review the birth experience. Suzi's experience goes to show that for a mother to feel truly fulfilled, whatever the circumstances, she must be heard, for she is profoundly guided by her instinctive silent voice, even if she doesn't recognize it.

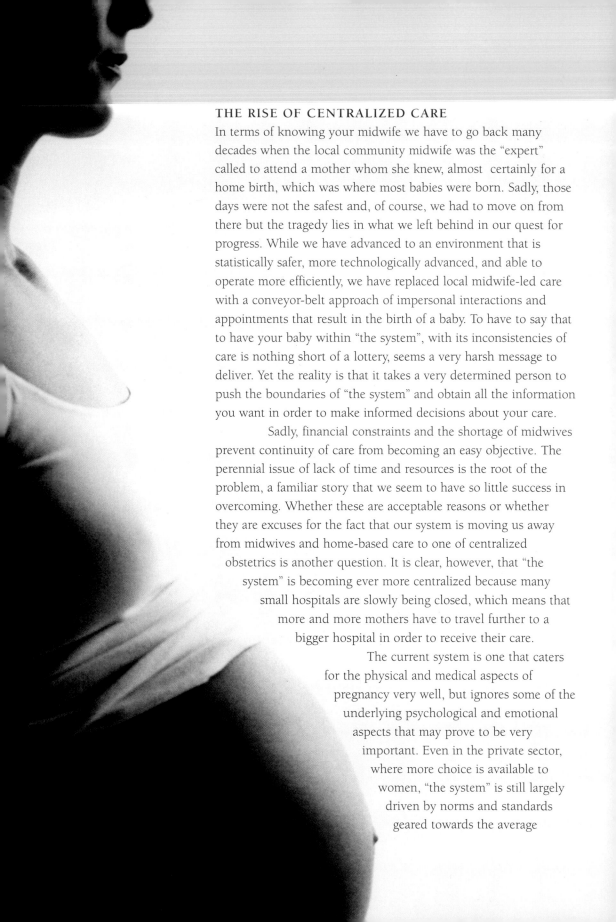

THE RISE OF CENTRALIZED CARE

In terms of knowing your midwife we have to go back many decades when the local community midwife was the "expert" called to attend a mother whom she knew, almost certainly for a home birth, which was where most babies were born. Sadly, those days were not the safest and, of course, we had to move on from there but the tragedy lies in what we left behind in our quest for progress. While we have advanced to an environment that is statistically safer, more technologically advanced, and able to operate more efficiently, we have replaced local midwife-led care with a conveyor-belt approach of impersonal interactions and appointments that result in the birth of a baby. To have to say that to have your baby within "the system", with its inconsistencies of care is nothing short of a lottery, seems a very harsh message to deliver. Yet the reality is that it takes a very determined person to push the boundaries of "the system" and obtain all the information you want in order to make informed decisions about your care.

Sadly, financial constraints and the shortage of midwives prevent continuity of care from becoming an easy objective. The perennial issue of lack of time and resources is the root of the problem, a familiar story that we seem to have so little success in overcoming. Whether these are acceptable reasons or whether they are excuses for the fact that our system is moving us away from midwives and home-based care to one of centralized obstetrics is another question. It is clear, however, that "the system" is becoming ever more centralized because many small hospitals are slowly being closed, which means that more and more mothers have to travel further to a bigger hospital in order to receive their care.

The current system is one that caters for the physical and medical aspects of pregnancy very well, but ignores some of the underlying psychological and emotional aspects that may prove to be very important. Even in the private sector, where more choice is available to women, "the system" is still largely driven by norms and standards geared towards the average woman. Of course, guidelines, protocols and policies need to be established in order to reduce mistakes and minimize any ill-resulting event and litigation. Many UK hospitals are introducing safe practice guidelines, thus allowing midwives increased flexibility when caring for women; we now need to accommodate the up-and-coming midwives in these training programmes.

Most women believe, albeit rather misguidedly, that "the system" will see them safely through this amazing time in their lives. Why should an intelligent woman think for one moment that "the system" would not have her best interests at heart? Being part of the system is one thing but making it work in your best interest is an entirely different kettle of fish. In many cases, women do not realize that they are dissatisfied with "the system" or aspects of it until a particular moment has passed. If only women could be made aware of potential frustrations at times when they can make proactive and informed decisions, based on their beliefs and expectations for pregnancy and birth. In this way, a woman would stand a chance of feeling that she has been empowered to make the right decision all along, rather than at 40 weeks, when she suddenly finds herself in an increasingly vulnerable situation over which she has very little control and very limited understanding.

It is common to see women subconsciously surrender to the system. Once they realize that they are not going to be able to establish a relationship with a midwife, and gain the trust of that person to help them achieve the birth of their dreams, they often will raise the white flag. Even those women who embark upon pregnancy and birth wanting to follow their instincts often end up conforming as they do not have the mental strength and resilience to persevere. And why should they? They are trying to concentrate on the baby inside them, not the minefield of obstetric bureaucracy.

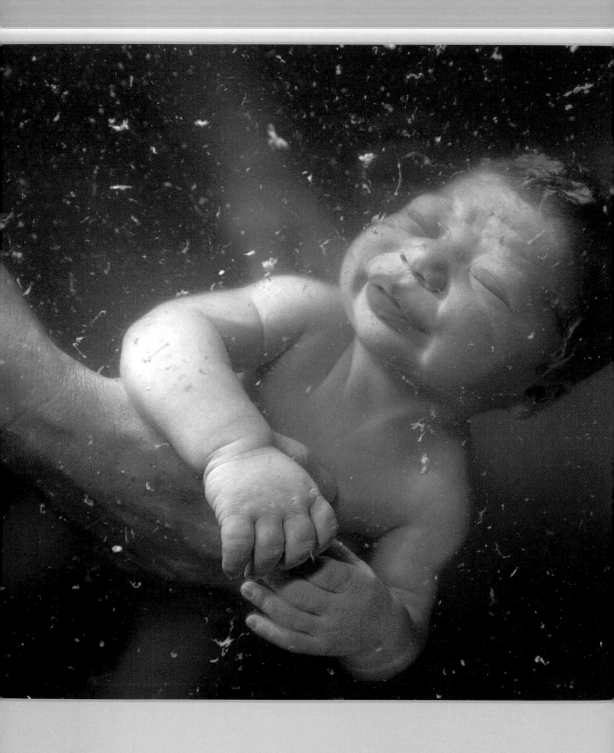

CHAPTER 3
Exploring the Options

✳ EXPLORING THE OPTIONS

Although we talk about three trimesters of pregnancy in the medical profession, I often think about pregnancy in terms of ten-week cycles. The first ten weeks is the cycle during which you discover you are pregnant, start to feel all the associated side-effects, and may even start to share the exciting news with friends and family. Weeks 10 to 20 will be those during which scans are performed, reassurances sought – and hopefully provided – and the news will disseminate if it hasn't already done so. It also may take you to the point when your pregnancy is showing physically and your baby is moving. Between weeks 20 and 30, the baby becomes viable and is growing steadily. This is also a time when many mothers will give up work – if they are able.

Once you reach the 31st week, you are in the home straight. At this last stage you may throw your hands up and wonder, "Who is out there for me? Who is going to be with me when I have my baby? What do I know, and what do I need to know?" Very often this is the time when a woman will start to seek out the alternative options available. In fact, the mothers who join an independent midwifery practice with their first pregnancies often do so at around 30 weeks, when their instincts are driving them to seek an alternative.

HOSPITAL BIRTHS

I really struggle to write about a healthy mother at term, in established labour, having her baby in hospital, especially the mother having her first baby. The reason being that the level of maternal satisfaction and fulfilment varies dramatically from hospital to hospital. In other words, it's a lottery. At this moment, due to the shortage of midwives and overstretched resources, nothing can be guaranteed for mothers approaching the birth of their babies. Sadly, not even the chosen hospital can be guaranteed, let alone whether you'll know your midwife.

Hospital births in the UK are full of "ifs". If you see a midwife more than once during your pregnancy – good. If a familiar, supportive midwife greets you when you arrive at the hospital in established labour – great. If that midwife listens to your wishes and expectations and reads and respects your birth plan – fantastic. If your midwife is supportive, encouraging and enables you to labour instinctively then your birth experience will, for sure, be the best it could be.

The usual disrespectful conveyor-belt approach to a woman's major life event is the reason why I became an independent midwife. An average hospital experience is one in which a woman will be "encouraged" to submit to a vaginal examination on or soon after her arrival. Food intake will be restricted. Should her contractions begin to decrease, an intravenous oxytocic infusion will be started to progress labour. If the labour is deemed too slow or the baby shows distress, a caesarean section is often the result.

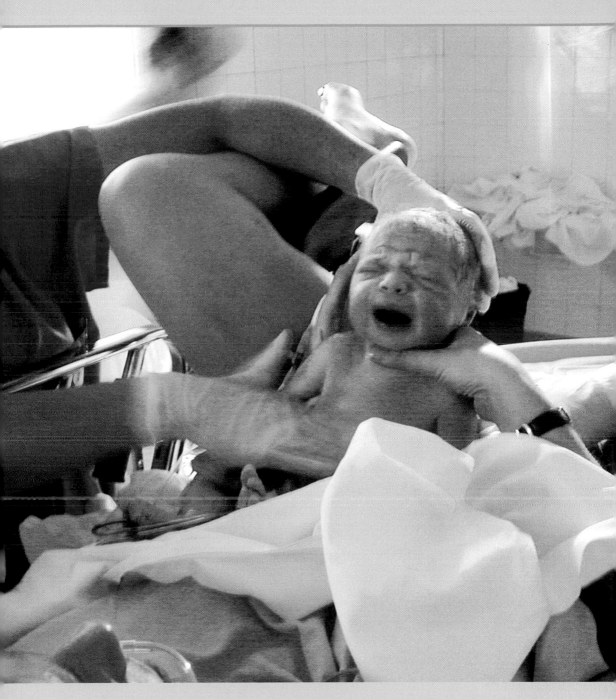

Most babies are born in hospital, and while it's perfectly
possible to give birth the way you would like to, you
need to be able to make sure all the team members have
your aims at heart.

Very recently I overheard two women talking. One was telling the other that her daughter was in hospital, in labour, but because her contractions were "only" every seven minutes, she must remain on the antenatal ward where her husband was not allowed. However, once she had progressed to contractions being every three minutes, then and only then would she be allowed to go to the delivery suite where her husband could join her. And this is the experience that the couple will remember forever!

BIRTHING CENTRES

There are many different options a woman can investigate in order to extricate herself from the routine mould. Some are found within and some outside "the system". One option that many women like to explore is that offered by birthing centres. These can be called midwife-led units, operating within the NHS, or they can be independent centres that are managed privately.

Midwife-led units tend to be linked to a mainstream hospital but are located independently, and are resourced by dedicated staff. They offer women the opportunity to birth their babies in a natural environment, without the pressure of technological intervention that tends to arise in the hospital. That said, the unit is usually in proximity to a hospital and, should a situation arise that requires immediate transfer, this is done quickly. Midwife-led units are a good step in the right direction, as their existence reaffirms the notion that midwives are best suited to handle normal pregnancies, and that the support of an obstetrician is only required when the abnormal occurs. Research has shown that less intervention increases the mutual benefit and satisfaction for both expectant mother and midwife. These units often are furnished along the lines of a "home-from-home", though hospitals vary greatly in their decorative capacities. Some simply hang curtains to conceal the equipment behind or maybe install a cheerful frieze around the walls. In more forward-thinking establishments, expectant mothers are accommodated during labour and birth in a truly domestic environment. This may include soft lighting, armchairs, a double bed, television, music and birthing pool – in fact, everything that will enable a woman to relax, concentrate and feel more encouraged to behave instinctively throughout the birth of her baby.

I am relieved and greatly encouraged by the increase in midwife-led units even though we still have far to go. The reality is that these hospital-based units tend to be under-resourced and, therefore, under-used. Although they are separate birthing centres, specializing in "natural deliveries", they are still part of "the system" and have to operate within the boundaries laid down. In other words, these units are constrained by hospital policy and are required to impose restrictions on the type of woman who is allowed to use them. If, for example, you are a first-time mother or already have had a caesarean section, it is unlikely that you would be considered suitable for the low-tech birth that these centres provide. A first-time mother may not be suitable because she may be deemed an "unknown entity" and, as such, her labour will be unpredictable. It would be nice to think that first-time mothers and mothers with potential complications, such as a previous caesarean section, could be accepted into such a unit instead of envisioning the worst-case scenario. In any event, doctors will not recommend or select midwife-led units or independent practices because they are in a convenient geographic location. Doctors will only recommend them if a mother is considered suitable to give birth in such a place. The principal criterion for qualification is a low-risk pregnancy.

One of the issues associated with midwife-led units is that the "just in case" scenario prevails. Those setting policy are still not looking at the boundaries of reasonableness. Yet they have only to look at birthing centre outcomes to see how much success can be derived from a non-interventionist approach. The audits are there to be scrutinized: an active birth in an environment in which a woman feels comfortable, coupled with a pre-existing expectant-mother-and-midwife relationship, produces more intervention-free, spontaneous vaginal births using less drugs. In other words, women are in control.

Our society has become so litigious that doctors will want to be secure in the knowledge that a woman is "qualified" to birth her baby in a midwifery-led unit.

I see this as a way forward and a safe option for an increasing number of women who wish to enjoy an instinctive birth. The challenge we face is how to make these centres more widely available when the system is driven by the fear of "what happens if?". Public sector centres cannot extend the boundaries and create pathways for change in the same way that those in the independent sector can. Attitudes within "the system" will only move forward as a result of sound research. Interestingly, the preference for woman-centred care and an intervention-free delivery is not just a message from parents-to-be, but also from many midwives, who experience much higher levels of job satisfaction from working in the birthing centres. The whole ethos is different, and to re-create this within a typical modern-day hospital (both physically and culturally), will pose a challenging task for many.

> **Labour is an activity that is undertaken by the mind and body; by interfering with one, the other will be affected.**

PRIVATE CENTRES

Private birthing centres are another option. These may or may not be located in proximity to a hospital and will endeavour to create a home-like environment for women in which they feel at ease and sufficiently relaxed to birth their babies instinctively. They have qualified midwives and occasionally doctors in attendance, all believing in a woman's ability to take control. Unfortunately in the UK, as yet we have all too few of these birthing centres. Once again, however, the level of non-interventionist births they produce proves that outcomes are significantly improved by more intimate and personal care, and when sufficient time is allowed for a woman to work with her body and instinct. Not only does this improve the outcome of the birth but, in many cases, the post-birth period when breastfeeding becomes established. A woman who has had a fulfilling birth experience is far more likely to succeed with breastfeeding.

HOME BIRTHS

The other alternative that seems obvious to some, and a crazy idea to others, is to birth your baby at home. A home birth provides the most natural and comforting environment in which to deliver. It allows a woman to act freely and as she feels fit, without the constraints imposed by hospitals. She can use the toilet and bath as necessary, she can help herself to food and drink as required, and up until a certain point in labour, she can be distracted from thinking about the discomfort of contractions by busying herself with things she has at home.

Once labour is fully established, many women find they need to be in a quiet place where they can concentrate on managing the contractions, almost allowing their body and mind to synchronize without unnecessary interference. A woman at home can adopt any position that makes her feel comfortable – using sofas, beds, cushions and birthing balls, if she wishes. More importantly, she can move around as much or as little as she wants. And, if she decides to use a birthing pool, she knows it will be available for her exclusive use as and when required.

An interesting phenomenon is that in many instances where women have been labouring very well at home, and coping steadily with the pain, they lose their contractions once they arrive at the hospital. It is well known that any movement imposed on a female animal while giving birth will stop labour, so it's no wonder that a woman will lose momentum upon transferring to the hospital.

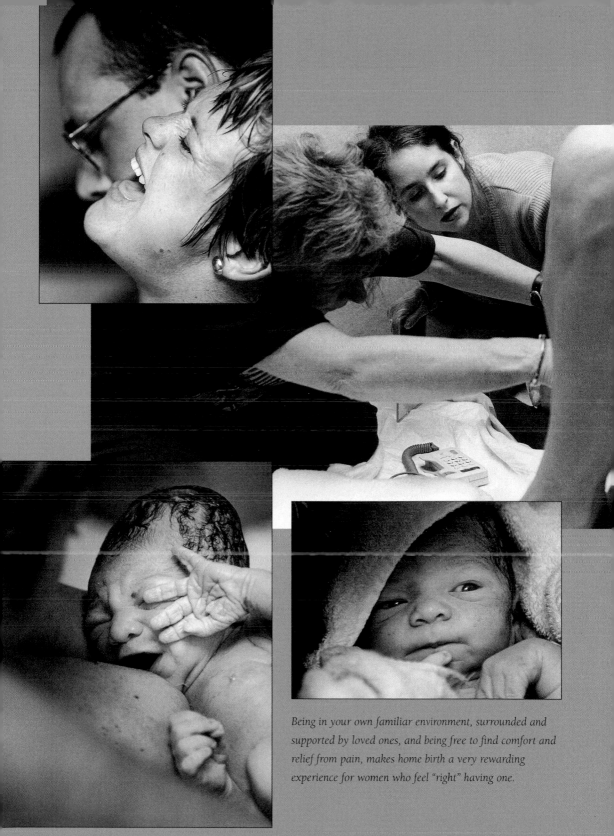

Being in your own familiar environment, surrounded and supported by loved ones, and being free to find comfort and relief from pain, makes home birth a very rewarding experience for women who feel "right" having one.

In Holland, over 30 percent of women birth their babies at home as this is considered the safest place for normal deliveries to take place. The Dutch maternity care system depends heavily on primary caregivers – midwives and general practitioners who are responsible for the care of women with low-risk pregnancies – while obstetricians are there to provide care for high-risk pregnancies.

WATER BIRTH

Those women opting for a water birth are making a wholly instinctive decision. Most women who choose to labour or birth their babies in water already have an affinity for using water as a method of pain relief or relaxation. Many of us when stressed enjoy relaxing in a warm bath with a few drops of lavender oil added. It is unsurprising then, that many pregnant women express the desire either to have a water birth in hospital, which sadly cannot be guaranteed, or hire a birth pool for a home water birth. Even with the choice of using water, some mothers once in established

A water birth is often the wished-for experience of women who are in touch with their instincts, but only if their instincts "tell them" that this is the case.

labour instinctively vacate the pool at some point before the birth, or decide not to use the pool at all.

Midwifery guidelines for hospital water births suggest that a labouring woman should resist entering the pool until her cervix has dilated to 5 cm! Unless we examine a woman, how can we possibly know if she is entering the pool at the "right" time (as per guidelines)? In my practice, with the pool filled once labour has begun and the temperature thermostatically controlled, I encourage my mothers only to enter the water when they feel they can no longer resist – whenever that might be!

MAKING A CHOICE

Deciding where to birth your baby is a very personal decision and one that may go through several iterations during the course of your pregnancy. Use the information and knowledge provided by this book to increase your instinctive awareness, and its ability to help you make decisions on where, when, and how to birth your baby. If you feel you want to deliver your baby at

I do firmly believe that instinctive birthing can take place in hospital, a midwife-led unit, or a birthing centre, just as much as at home, if that is where a mother chooses to have her baby.

Jackie, a delightfully well-informed client, is about to deliver her second baby. Her first labour and birth were totally hospital managed, which was not what she wanted, and she was even denied immediate bonding with her newborn as the baby was swiftly transferred to the special care baby unit because she was cold. Her husband, on the other hand, still believes that every procedure was necessary and thanks heaven they were in hospital.

Jackie is desperate to have her second baby at home, but her husband refuses even to discuss the issue. He has been deeply influenced by his first birth experience and, never having had the opportunity to discuss or explore his feelings – something men by and large are not very good at – I'm sure his reaction is based purely on love and wanting the best for his wife and new baby.

home – so be it. In my experience, the most wonderful, relaxed and instinctive births have been those that took place in the comfort and security of my expectant mothers' own homes. Most of my labouring women, safe in the security and comfort of their personal surroundings, feel free to use their own devices to cope with their labours, and although I am there to assist them as they wish, my role often becomes that of quiet bystander. It is not easy to achieve this in a hospital where inevitably noise, strange faces and a clinical environment are the norm. Home birth, however, is not for everyone.

Ultimately, you may be left with your GP as the only potential source of information you have before entering "the system". Of course, in many countries, the GP or his or her equivalent is part of "the system", but that does not mean he or she cannot provide information on all the available options. Let's face it: once you arrive in the hospital to be booked in, what would make the hospital think you would like to explore alternative options? You are pregnant, excited, and the staff there are just going to go along with that excitement. At this point, the likelihood of a mother being advised of alternative options and thus referring herself out is negligible.

Your decision also may be heavily influenced by your partner. While the changing male role is to be applauded, it should not be discounted that, generally speaking, most men feel more comfortable in a hospital. I have often seen women keen to explore alternative options, but due to the influence of their partners, decide to opt for a hospital birth. In many ways it is natural for a man to feel safer in a hospital environment – it is "officially sanctioned", everyone he knows has had their babies there, it's got plenty of equipment and doctors. It is often a combination of love and concern for their partners along with peer pressure that makes many men feel that hospital is the best option.

However, the more a man appreciates the normality of pregnancy, labour, and birth, the more he will, in turn, help his expectant partner to make an informed decision with which both parties are comfortable. Only through understanding the normal birth process and being reassured of its safety can a man truly support his partner's choices.

WHERE TO FIND ADVICE

Identifying appropriate information and finding the right level of knowledge will differ from individual to individual. In the UK, we cannot guarantee that the midwife who cares for a couple before the birth will be present at the birth itself. This can be very disappointing for a couple who start to build a relationship with "their" midwife and see her as part of the team. Thus the more prepared a couple are and the more knowledge they have, the more they can be totally involved in their birth, irrespective of where it takes place and who is present. It's important to seek information outside "the system". Independent birthing classes, for example, will greatly enhance the probability of a good birth experience – no matter where the birth takes place.

*   Sandra, the mother of a lively daughter born in an uncomplicated delivery in the hospital, was expecting twins. Initially, as her pregnancy advanced healthily, Sandra felt that she could look forward to a normal, uncomplicated delivery. However, many of her friends, who were also having babies at this time, began to relate stories of problems that they had encountered at the hospital where Sandra was planning to give birth. Some talked of serious staff shortages and their having to labour alone for long periods of time. Others said their call bells took a very long time to be answered. Alarmed by these stories, but still trusting in her instinct to choose the safest birth for her babies, Sandra reluctantly decided to have her babies by elective caesarean section. In this way she felt she could ensure that sufficient health care professionals necessary for a safe outcome would be there on the day, and, indeed, Jack and Tom were delivered safely and soundly.

One of the underlying reasons that we have become so accepting of the conveyor belt approach to maternity care is our exposure to childbirth in the media. These days there is more information available on pregnancy and childbirth than at any other time – magazines, books, television, video, the Internet and even some medical research papers are in the public domain. Any modern-day woman exposed to television or magazines, would think that lying on a bed in a brightly lit room, with an intravenous drip in place to accelerate her labour, monitors bleeping continuously, surrounded by an array of hospital personnel giving instructions on when and how to push, is quite a natural way to give birth. Birth is constantly shown in a high-tech environment in which a team of medical specialists are on tap to whisk the baby away to start suctioning the mucus and cleaning him up. What is there to make us think that our personal experiences could or should be any different? Where is the woman giving birth on her own in water, completely unassisted and uninterrupted by anyone except maybe her husband, who gives her reassuring words or touches her from time to time? Where is the woman who is in hospital on a couch, kneeling or squatting down, birthing her baby and then holding him and gazing at him intently for a good few minutes before that magical moment ends with baby checks, etc.? Why in every birth scene on TV is there a group of doctors and nurses, beeping machines, and a woman lying down? Birth was never meant to be like this.

Even when working within "the system", I do my best to give couples increased control through imparting knowledge and information, and by helping them do what their instincts direct. I explain the way in which "the system" operates and prepare them for any potential consequences of the events that they may encounter. Specifically, I discuss the possibility that the hospital will want to do an internal examination of the labouring woman, and even make her lie on a bed to monitor her progress. I inform partners that their wives may not necessarily need to succumb to internal examinations unless they so desire or there is a sound obstetric reason for this intrusion. Likewise, if a woman wants to give birth in an upright position or to walk around during labour, I encourage her husband to remember this, and to be strong with the hospital staff if unnecessarily prolonged monitoring is undertaken during advancing labour.

MAKING YOUR VOICE HEARD

It takes quite a proactive and assertive person, who is listening to her instincts and searching for alternative options, to explore the possibility of any independent bodies outside the system. This is even truer when it's a first-time mother who may meet quite forceful objections from her obstetrician or midwife, her partner, and even members of her close circle who just would not contemplate challenging the status quo. That said, there are many organizations that will support a woman's dreams of an empowered birth based on informed decisions. These organizations can offer great support for women looking to achieve the birth of their choice.

Following your instinct, however, does not necessarily mean that you have to eschew routine. Many women heeding their instincts are led directly down routine's path. A woman may be attuned to all her innermost feelings, perfectly at home in her body and the developing life within her, yet feels that in the case of a deviation from the norm, a caesarean section might be the best option for her and her baby. I know plenty of women who, having found themselves in an abnormal situation, such as multiple pregnancy, or even a breech presentation, and having sought the facts and questioned caregivers, made an informed decision that they would prefer a caesarean. Questioned weeks and again years after the event, they still feel that they did the best for their babies, and that they had successful birthing experiences. Their instincts were just as strong as first-time mothers who chose to birth their babies in a pool at home. The solution for each woman was different, but the woman felt in control and the outcome was positive.

This book is not looking to discourage women from using what is available to them in terms of technology and the standard practices in hospitals. However, I do encourage you to listen to your body, heed what your instinct tells you and, if necessary, question the routine procedures of "the system". "Why do I need this early scan?" "Do I really understand what this may or may not be doing to my baby?" "Will I be able to deal with the results of the scan and, if not, why have it?" "Is my partner in agreement?" Questioning routine is something that starts when your baby is a growing fetus and continues throughout your life as a parent. The practice of understanding what is being provided and recommended by "the system" – whether healthcare, schooling or sport or leisure-time activity – is an important one, as it allows you, the parent, to make an informed decision, one you are much less likely to regret further down the line. From experience, I know that how and by whom a mother is counselled regarding any aspect of pregnancy but especially a deviation from the norm, will directly influence her ability to touch base with her instincts and thus her potential for a better result.

The best birthing experiences are ones where women feel looked after but also part of the decision-making process. Help is at hand if needed but unless there's a problem, the labouring woman should be left to deliver as her body directs.

My message in conclusion to this chapter is that you do not have to birth your baby outside the system to be instinctive. As long as they are cushioned by feelings of safety and security, all mothers-to-be, even those expecting their first babies, will always make a safe decision about where and how they will labour and birth their babies. Your instincts are with you wherever you go, they may become undermined within the confinement of hospital walls, but they are still there, ready to be heard. You will have to be more assertive and more confident of your instinct within the system, but that is no reason to ignore it. Your baby is communicating with you at all times; listen to his voice in whatever shape it may come.

Having a good birthing experience, one that is based on you making the decisions and being supported by a sensitive caregiver, will make you want to share it with everyone you meet! It is only natural that this will mean that other women will be interested and think "Oh, I did not realize birthing could be like that." It only takes a small nucleus of people to start a new wave of thinking. If we can start to inspire women to pursue the birth experience of their dreams, maybe this will have the more universal effect of changing our approach to childbirth, and reverting to one where the instinct of the woman is the overriding guide and driving force.

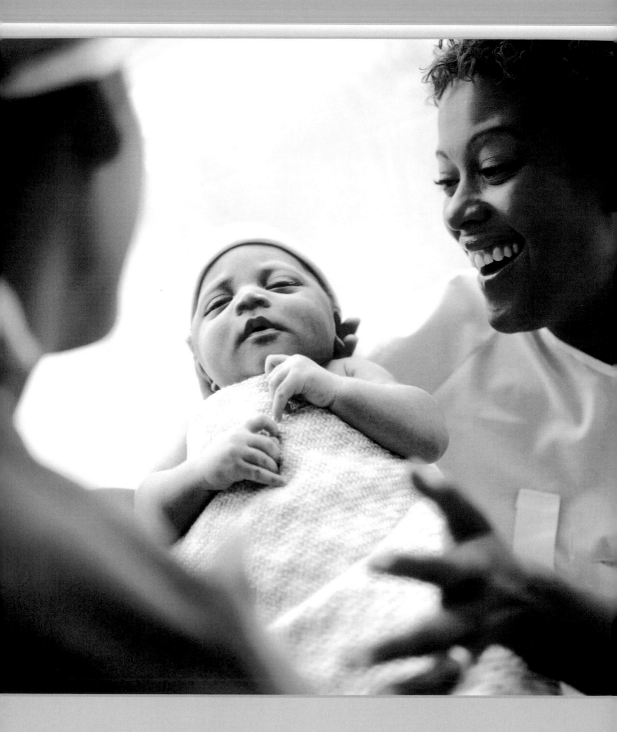

CHAPTER 4
Care Through Partnership

✳ CARE THROUGH PARTNERSHIP

Care through partnership means finding people within midwifery or obstetrics with whom you not only seek professional advice and care, but with whom you can build a trusting relationship during pregnancy. The objective of care through partnership is that you feel that decisions are made jointly, and that childbirth becomes an experience on which you have worked collaboratively. The person responsible for your care will spend time getting to know you and your partner, listening to your dreams, your aspirations and any fears or concerns. He or she will help you to obtain information that is meaningful to you, and encourage you to take an active role in decision-making, particularly so you can make informed choices. As a result, if an unforeseen situation arises requiring a decision, you can be confident that your carer understands your aspirations for birth and personal circumstances, and will help you and your partner to make a wise choice.

CHOOSING YOUR PARTNERS

Care through partnership does not necessarily imply a private obstetrician or an independent midwife. It can be sought within the public sector just as much as outside of it. That being said, the state-funded system may not be able to provide this type of care as it involves the mother knowing her practitioner, and being confident that he or she will be able to attend the birth of her baby. In the UK, we struggle desperately with resources, especially those within the community. As hospital birthing has increasingly become the status quo, there seems to be a reluctant acceptance among women that they cannot expect to know who is going to support them throughout pregnancy and birth. Expectant mothers tend to accept that when they turn up at the hospital on the day or night of their labours, they will be met and cared for by whoever is on duty at the time.

If you work with an independent midwife, you'll be able to call her morning, noon or night, and she'll assist you with your birth. Working with the same individual enables you to build a trusting relationship, and to feel special and important. Knowing that the midwife who has provided you with prenatal care will be present at your baby's birth, and subsequently will care for you both following the birth, has a very positive impact on confidence levels. Such a relationship generally produces a vaginal birth with less intervention and less pain relief. Moreover, you will be directly involved in your pattern of care and encouraged to understand and listen to your instincts. Research has established again and again that when mothers know and trust their midwives, birthing outcomes are often far more successful. Personal experience has also shown that this type of care through partnership will increase a mother's awakening awareness to trust her body and her instincts.

In contrast to an obstetrician, who can refuse to care for a pregnant woman, for example, if he or she feels that a patient is making unreasonable demands or those he or she cannot safely fulfil such as a water birth, a midwife is legally bound by a duty of care.

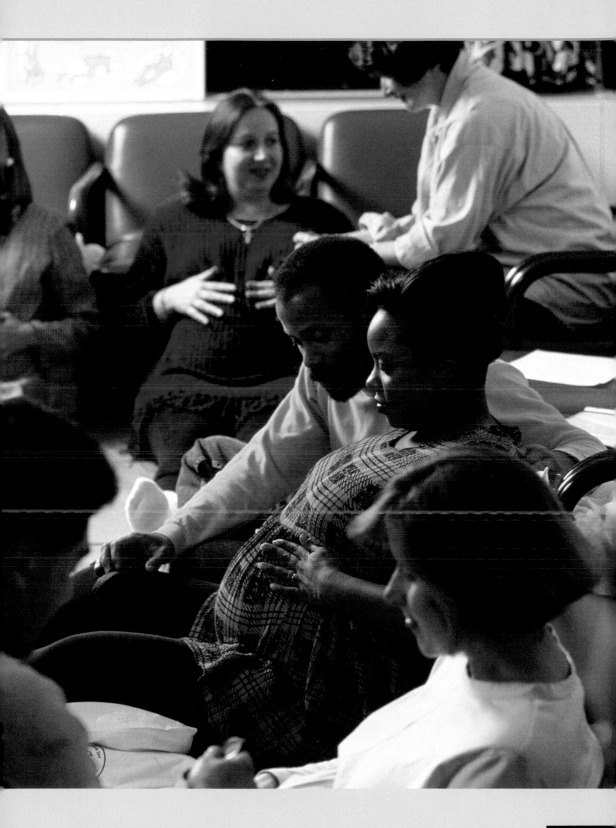

Her code of practice and midwifery rules bind her to become the health professional responsible for an expectant mother, irrespective of whether or not she agrees with the selected birthing location, and providing it's within her sphere of practice.

While the cost of an independent midwife may be prohibitive for some, I have known many couples sell cars or windfall shares, or take out bank loans to cover the cost of a service that they deem to be an integral part of their pregnancy and birth. And it's not surprising they make this sacrifice as the relationship between an independent midwife and a pregnant woman is very special. It is special because they have chosen each other. They have agreed to form a partnership over the next few months and have to work to a set of mutual aspirations. Independent midwives aim to provide a level of care that is seamless. Women under their care will feel they are receiving continuous support, regardless of the situation and location in which they birth their babies.

INFORMATION PROVIDER

All midwives believe that pregnancy and birth is a normal, biological event in a healthy woman's life. In order that the expectant mother in her care is given the necessary information to make informed choices, a midwife takes time at each antenatal visit, often in the woman's home, to listen to and appreciate her as an individual with individual feelings. A midwife also takes responsibility for equipping an expectant mother with knowledge and information at the depth and pace she requests – not every book, article or website is right for every woman. Each woman will approach pregnancy in a different way, and thus her appetite for knowledge will differ. Some women prefer practical books; some like factual, research-based books; others request holistic, spiritual books, and a few may just want to read the humorous books. Likewise, television may or may not be an effective medium to suggest to a mother-to-be, depending on how much she wants to see, and how aspects of pregnancy and childbirth that are presented on television compare to her own personal perceptions and beliefs.

It is widely recognized that midwives, not obstetricians, are the "experts" as far as normal pregnancies and births are concerned.

Knowing which media to suggest to a woman is an important part of care through partnership, as this will influence how the expectant mother builds her own picture of pregnancy and childbirth. Ask a newly pregnant woman the typical pregnancy-related questions such as: "Where do you want to have your baby?", "How do you want to have your baby?", "What pain relief do you want?" and most will reply: "In the

✻ Lucy, an American mother, pregnant with her first baby, decided early on to engage the services of a private obstetrician, in keeping with the traditional American pattern of care, and believing that by doing so her instincts would be respected. It soon became apparent after attending routine antenatal visits that Lucy's expectations and hopes for her pregnancy and birth differed greatly from those held by her obstetrician. Once she became acutely aware of the constraints within the general system of care, she sought my services as an independent midwife. The partnership of care between Lucy, her husband and me grew stronger as the weeks passed. With the full support of her husband, plans were put in place for Lucy to birth her baby at home. Her obstetrician remained somewhat sceptical, and tried to persuade Lucy to opt for the "home from home" birthing room at the hospital. Needless to say, I fully supported Lucy, encouraging her to listen to and respect her instinct to birth her baby at home.

When Lucy was well advanced in active labour, she requested a vaginal examination as she felt the information derived from this – how much her cervix was effaced and how far down the birth canal her baby had progressed – might encourage her in coping with her increasingly powerful contractions. During the examination, however, her waters ruptured and they, unfortunately, were meconium stained. This event can be a reason for transfer to the hospital and in this case I felt that such a move was desirable and Lucy agreed.

Our transfer was seamless and Lucy continued to labour without interference once she had settled in and familiarized herself with her new surroundings. Support was on hand with technology readily available should the need arise. In her birth plan, Lucy had expressed that she did not want to be made to lie down and that she wanted to be actively involved in all decision-making. I was able to support her in those wishes when she was at her most vulnerable. After a two-hour, healthy second stage, Lucy birthed her baby in a squatting position, which she had instinctively adopted. Her obstetrician quietly observed the birth and later thanked Lucy for affording him the opportunity to witness such a beautiful, normal birth. Within two hours of the birth, Lucy had quietly bathed with her baby and returned home. She had experienced an empowered and fulfilling birth and has already said that, all being well, she will definitely seek to birth her future babies at home.

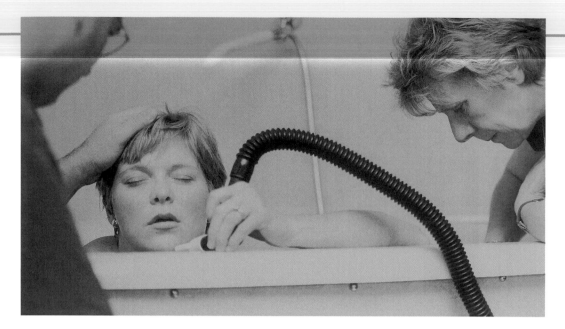

Everyone present at a birth – be they intimately connected with the mother or an attendant – should be helping the mother to work with her instincts and to birth her baby in her own time.

hospital, with every pain relieving drug available!". In her ignorance I might add, as she has nothing more than media images and a low level of information upon which to base her knowledge. She even may request an elective caesarean section, having been advised, usually by her obstetrician, that it is extremely simple to have a spinal anaesthetic, a few days of antibiotic cover, and more importantly, an exact date in your diary when you will become a mother. How tempting is that for a professional woman who often knows very little about childbirth except that it's painful!

THE IDEAL FORM OF CARE

At the initial appointment, which is usually lengthy, a midwife will compile detailed and comprehensive notes, covering the woman's general health and wellbeing, obstetric history, medical history, and both hers and the father's family history, if available. Within the notes, which the expectant mother has for safekeeping, is a section in which both she and her partner can explore and document their feelings, if they wish, as to the type of birth desired – home or hospital, why they've chosen a midwife, their relationship with their own mothers, and how they feel about becoming parents.

Intelligent mothers do not make unwise or unsafe decisions regarding their own or their baby's safety. If a woman has an adverse medical or obstetric history that will limit her birth choice – for example if she has insulin-dependent diabetes – she welcomes the fact that her midwife will support her safely through the system as her advocate and friend. If a woman has a baby in hospital, she will be delivered by other attendants but her midwife will become her birth supporter, sitting with her and offering quiet reassurance.

Once documentation is completed, a woman or the couple and their midwife will embark on one of life's most incredible experiences, pregnancy and birth. Together they will embrace the normality or cope with any deviation that may occur, only saying goodbye 4-6 weeks after the birth.

An independent midwife's approach to childbirth is the traditional one – a pregnancy is normal and healthy until proved otherwise – even if previous pregnancies have been complicated.

WORKING WITHIN "THE SYSTEM"

As you progress throughout your pregnancy, your instincts will help you to find the level and type of care that allows you to feel safe and confident. Hopefully, the person responsible for your care will make you feel special, respect your aspirations, and encourage you to participate in decisions based on information and choice. While private or independent care may afford a more intimate relationship with a midwife or obstetrician, it is not out of your reach to work towards a similar partnership within "the system". If you are allocated a community midwife, and she is part of a pooled team, why not try to meet as many different team members as possible, in order that you can identify a couple of midwives who make you feel most comfortable? By attending their clinics and prenatal classes you will be able to develop a closer relationship with them and hopefully work together towards your pregnancy and birthing objectives. Guaranteeing that a particular midwife is there at the time of birth may not be a realistic expectation within the current system, and for many women this may be a source of disappointment. Yet there is a positive aspect in that you have built a trusting relationship with some of your caregivers, who have helped you to increase your self-confidence and to take an active role in the decision-making process.

The relationships I developed with the mothers I cared for were trusting, patient, and lasting. Treasured cards, photos and messages that I have received from mothers over the years are a constant reminder of the humble part I played in their life's experiences. I am so proud of the women I cared for and the approach they took to making informed decisions, using their instincts to make themselves and their partners more empowered to fulfil their desired birth.

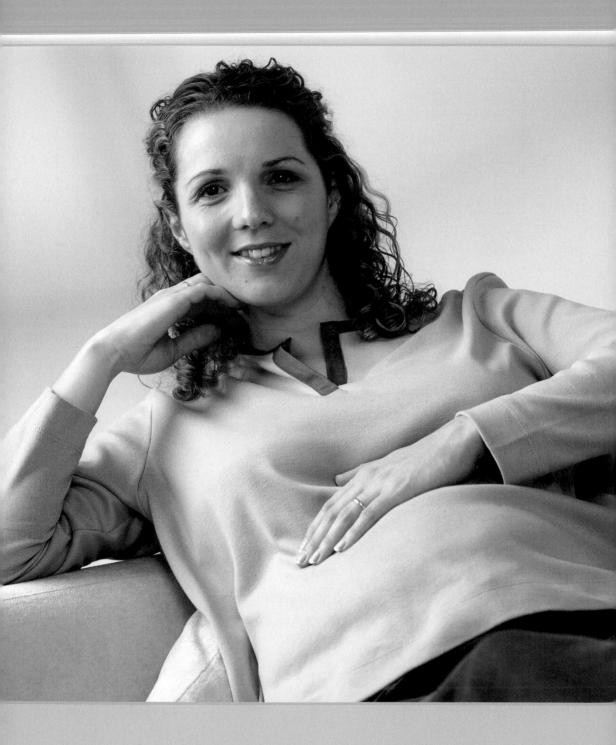

CHAPTER 5
Reawakening Your Instincts

✳ REAWAKENING YOUR INSTINCTS

Centuries ago, a woman's menstrual cycle often tended to follow that of the lunar cycles. This is not surprising as the clock was not part of a woman's daily routine, and her contact with the stars and other heavenly bodies was greater than ours is today. Our forebears were much more aware of the influences brought about by planetary movements; after all, the sun and moon ruled their days and nights. Moreover, they could more clearly see the stars and the moon, as these were not obscured by the tall buildings, artificial lighting and air pollution that are so prevalent today. Often women would come together around the time that they were menstruating and look after each other. They would keep very much to themselves – sometimes in purpose-built or special private sanctuaries – and the men in the group would respect this as a time in the month when women should be left alone. Men were afraid of women's ability to bear children, and tried to strengthen their own self-esteems by regarding menstruating women as unclean and separating them from the group. Menstruation and childbirth were regarded as women's mysteries and were generally taboo subjects.

Certain of these attitudes were still around in my day, as they were in my mother's and grandmother's. Women and girls growing up did not talk about their bodies or anything to do with the functioning of the human body. My grandmother used to refer to periods as the "poorly time". My sister used to refer to it as "the curse". That shows you how becoming a woman was perceived. Women were not encouraged to be in tune with their bodies and to celebrate their fertility, but simply to put up with the inconvenience. This also was the approach to pregnancy and childbirth, which were perceived as experiences to be endured as part of the female role.

There is a significant change happening now. Girls are much more aware of their bodies, of who they are, and how their bodies function. They are exposed to biology studies that explain how the body works and how reproduction occurs. And whereas in the past couples waited until they were in their 20s and married before having intercourse and, hopefully, producing babies, many of today's girls and boys are engaging in sexual activities before they are 16, and parenthood is the last thing on their minds! (Although youngsters are more informed than ever, many are still sexually ignorant.)

TUNING IN TO YOUR BODY

We would like to believe that as girls mature and become women, they are taking more control of their bodies. Obviously the use of contraceptive devices is commonplace, not just to prevent pregnancy but also to deter infection. But women are starting to become interested in something more than just physical control – greater intimacy with their bodies, on an emotional and, in some cases, a spiritual level.

Many women today want to learn how, in addition to the physical and biological interactions that may be manipulated by drugs, their menstrual cycles and

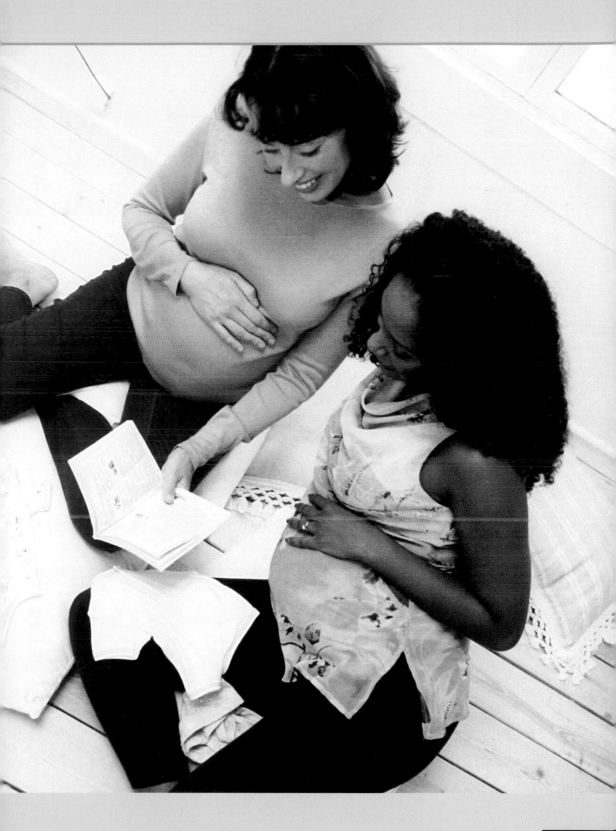

fertility levels can be affected. How many times do we hear about couples who have given up on having a baby after years of fertility treatment, suddenly finding they've become pregnant once treatment is abandoned? How much has been written about how the diet and specific foods may boost our fertility levels? How often is it claimed that the "hazards" of modern life reduce fertility? How much are we starting to learn about the patterns of ovulation and the possibility that there are planetary influences that may well affect the timing of conception? In fact, only recently, it has been reported that a fertile woman may ovulate more than once in her menstrual cycle. The world has become a more informed place and because of it our attitudes are changing.

Complementary medicine is also having an increasingly strong influence on our approach to seeking treatment and greater understanding of our bodies. Homeopaths,

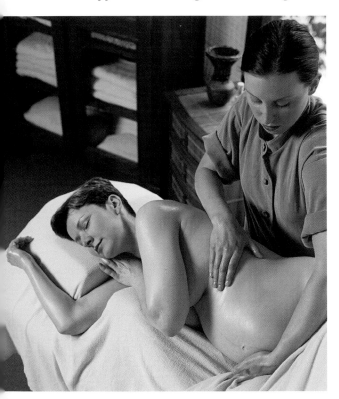

Many women, both in an attempt to conceive and to ensure a healthy pregnancy, prefer to eschew drug treatment in favour of more "alternative" therapies, which are less invasive of their bodies.

reflexologists, aromatherapists, naturopaths, acupuncturists and Chinese herbalists all can offer advice and therapies to help a woman better regulate her menstrual cycle, and possibly improve her fertility. Such therapists look at the situation from a holistic angle; they try to understand a woman's lifestyle, diet, relationships and other influencing factors that may be affecting the ebbs and flows of her cycle. Slowly but surely doctors, too, are beginning to accept that there might be other ways to promote wellbeing, and increasing numbers, albeit still too few, are practicing both conventional and complementary medicine.

Increasing numbers of women are becoming more comfortable reading and talking about their bodies, and even sharing this information with their partners. Learning to understand your menstrual cycles, when you ovulate and the physical and emotional changes that take place within your body at that time, allows you to become more in tune with your body and more aware of your fertile periods, however predictable or unpredictable they may be. This is a very positive approach when it comes to trying for a baby, as it means you can have a deeper understanding about what constitutes healthy conception and pregnancy.

On a more spiritual level, there are many ways of becoming more connected with the inner you. Yoga and Pilates have very positive effects on the mind and body but also have been known to nurture the spirit. The ability to take some time to concentrate on your breathing and to focus on the movement and the response your body is giving to that movement teaches you to listen to what your body is telling you at that time. This is like a meditation through movement, and is an effective first step towards listening to your body and hearing the messages it communicates.

The thoughts, images or ideas each woman uses to visualize in childbirth will differ from woman to woman, but the objective is to focus on images that make a woman feel safe, comfortable and happy.

Meditation is a less tangible but stronger form of concentration; it uses the mind and teaches you to focus on your inner core and reach for universal knowledge. It also creates a discipline by which you are able to remove the unnecessary thoughts and worries of everyday life, and thus has a powerful remedial effect on the body.

There is a strong emotional connection between the mind and the body, so even if you focus more on one than the other, you will probably feel a positive impact at both levels. Visualization is another effective technique that focuses your mind on your aspirations and desires. This is a great tool to use at many times in your life, especially when you are facing a challenge or seeking mental strength. Focusing on happy thoughts or comforting images and memories helps your mind to create more positive thoughts and this in turn will affect your behaviour. Visualization has proven very successful during labour, as women instinctively in tune with their bodies can imagine their babies coming down the birth canal and starting to emerge.

Tuning in to your body is an important part of pregnancy. Some aspects will hit you hard, such as the more physical signs of early pregnancy – the morning sickness, your enlarging breasts, fatigue and constipation. These are common in pregnancy and most women are aware of them and, to a certain extent, are able to manage them through adjusting their diets, making time for relaxation, and, occasionally, taking medication. There are, however, other aspects of pregnancy that will be less obvious, especially those that relate to your mental and emotional outlook.

It also is important to know your strengths and weaknesses; you need to understand what is and is not acceptable to you as an individual, and how far you can go with your body. With your first baby you may have little or no idea of your limits but the process of discovery should be magical and wholly empowering. You are inside your body and you are the one who knows it best. Familiarity with your instinct is so much easier once you understand your body.

INSTINCT

When I read through some of the scores of books available on the subject of pregnancy and childbirth, I always feel that one core message is lacking. That is the message about instinct: understanding what it is, how it exists within each and every one of us, and how it can be accessed and used effectively for pregnancy and childbirth. Instinct, according to Collins' Dictionary, can be defined as "inborn intuitive power" – in other words it is a tool with which we came equipped into this world.

How can we expect to feel confident about pregnancy and birth if we do not know how to use our primal instinct?

Instinct lies within you and you may experience it as a physical, emotional or psychological feeling.

During early pregnancy and sometimes throughout its term, what we call nature often provides our bodies with direction as to what it needs in order to nourish a baby and sustain a healthy pregnancy. Quite commonly, food and drink that you consumed as part of your daily routine, such as a lunchtime piece of pizza or a cup of coffee in the morning, will no longer be palatable. Suddenly, you no longer have a taste for those items in your diet that are not so good for you during pregnancy. Some may even make you feel physically sick. On the other hand, there may be foods that you suddenly feel a great desire to eat, and these may be derived from food groups that your body is lacking. Very often the cravings that arise during pregnancy are linked to foods in which a mother's diet is deficient.

In a similar vein, particularly in early pregnancy, your body may give you very strong signals that it needs more rest, reminding you of the new life developing within you. Many women feel extremely tired during the early stages of pregnancy, as hormones bring about changes in the body and it starts to work for two instead of one. If you are in tune with your body, you should succumb to the need for more rest. You also may find your dreams become very vivid and quite different from any you have had in the past. Your mind is also adapting to the fact that you are pregnant, and dreaming allows your subconscious to express itself and tune in to the changes taking place within your body.

There is a difference, however, between following your instinct and following your body even though the two are very closely interwoven. Both are about ignoring the day-to-day challenges, duties and expectations in order to discover what is going on within, but bodily needs are linked more to your physical state and instinct has more to do with your mental state. The latter is subconscious knowledge that you have and may never have tapped into or even realized exists.

An example of your body "talking" is the overwhelming and often unexpected tiredness often associated with the early weeks of pregnancy. Many women are unaware of the dramatic changes that are taking place within their newly pregnant bodies. Believing quite rightly that pregnancy is normal and healthy, they refuse to succumb to the often debilitating tiredness, endeavouring instead to continue their normal day-to-day routines without realizing that to do so is to exacerbate the early pregnancy symptoms of nausea, vomiting and lack of concentration.

Human instinct, on the other hand, can force your body to perform a certain way in an attempt to ensure your survival. Consider the notion of fight or flight: when an adverse or fearful situation presents itself, do you freeze or do you run? The reaction you follow is totally instinctive. Suppose, for example, when driving, you suddenly see a car in front of you and realize you are going to hit it. Do you swerve or do you brake? Instinct will be the driving force behind your decision as it is unlikely that the rational side of your brain has time to calculate the logical response. In other words, the situation arises too fast for the conscious brain to decide, so an immediate response is made from somewhere far deeper, a response that will always promote self-preservation. Sir Robert Winston, in his book *Human Instinct* provides an interesting insight into the way in which instinctive decisions are made, triggered by a biochemical reaction from within a specific area of the brain. He says: "This primal emotion, to advance or retreat, is triggered so fast that it precedes all conscious thought and awareness."

Janice was in advanced pregnancy when she informed her hospital-assigned midwife at an antenatal visit that she really didn't want to have any internal examinations during her labour, if at all possible. The midwife was bemused and advised her that there was no other way of assessing her progress. During her labour, Janice felt increasingly vulnerable as she was continually pressured to comply with hospital protocol and to have examinations that she found both uncomfortable and invasive.

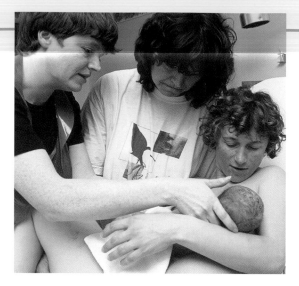

Instinct may lead you to have your baby in hospital – if that is where you think you will "feel" the safest. This is usually the case with first-time mothers, who generally require the full experience of birth to become fully acquainted with their innermost feelings.

The type of instinct I refer to throughout this book is not a result of a physiological interaction, but it is something in each and every one of us that is always present but deep within our very being. It is a knowing instinct and is what could be defined as "inborn knowing power". During pregnancy and childbirth, this knowing power is not what "tells" you your body is tired – that is a physical feeling your body has and should be respected – it is more about learning to listen to what you feel is the correct path to take or a decision that is right for you and your baby. In fact, you may not be aware that you are making conscious decisions as you follow where your instinct leads.

As I mentioned earlier, it is quite common for first-time mothers, around the 30th week of pregnancy or in the "home straight" as I describe it, to instinctively begin to evaluate who is out there for them, to guide and nurture them through the final phase of pregnancy and birth. Up to that moment, most first-time mothers have gone along with what "the system" has to offer, so why do they now begin to question and attempt to seek out an alternative – their instincts. Unfortunately, the majority of first-time mothers are unaware of the possible alternatives, and so in an attempt to be in control of their labours and births, they write a birth plan – only to find out that it doesn't comply with the guidelines/protocol/policies of their chosen hospitals.

In countries where a hospital birth is actively encouraged by those in authority, a woman who decides to birth her baby at home is responding to her instinct that this is the safest place for her and her baby. While it may be seen as an irrational decision, based on a personal whim, for such a woman, however, this decision feels very rational and very safe. Her instinct is driving her to act against the status quo, but she feels confident that this is the right decision for her and her baby unless an unforeseen problem arises.

Without realizing it, from the first moments you learn you are pregnant, you will act instinctively to protect your child. You will actually hold your tummy to shield your baby – an embrace that encompasses you both. Pregnant women often become more conservative in their outlooks, and may develop aversions to activities that they previously deemed risk-free. Their instincts are making them very protective of their

✳   Returning from her holiday, Helen was able to confirm that her long-standing dream of another baby had been granted, and she was six weeks' pregnant. Overjoyed, she quickly shared the news with her friends and family. Later that same week, Helen awoke with the feeling the baby had died. She couldn't explain the reason for this feeling but wanted to have an early scan just to reassure herself that she was being unnecessarily paranoid. On arrival at the hospital Helen was asked whether she had experienced any abdominal pain or bleeding. Helen said "No" but that she just didn't feel the baby was healthy. She was told she could book a scan for the following week but since there were no physical symptoms, she could not have the scan that day. Leaving the hospital, Helen tried to rationalize her emotions. She reasoned that up to that point, she had been acting impulsively and that there was no reason for her to be rushing to the hospital at the slight feeling of doubt. Moreover, she had an important day ahead and that her reaction to the baby's wellbeing may have been a manifestation of nerves related to another situation. She returned home and told her husband how silly she felt and that she would try to be more relaxed in future. She did try to put the negative thoughts behind her and carried on as usual waiting for her 12 weeks scan.

     Four weeks later Helen noticed some slight bleeding. She went straight to her GP who advised a trip to the hospital. As the sonographer placed the probe on her abdomen, Helen knew that her fears were about to be confirmed. The smile on the sonographer's face disappeared and she gazed intensely at the screen. Helen asked if the baby was alive. The sonographer replied that there was a sac and a baby, but no heartbeat. The baby had developed to just over six weeks' gestation. Helen assured the sonographer that her dates were correct; it was optimistic to think she could be wrong. Two days later the miscarriage was complete; a baby who was there one minute had gone the next.

     Looking back, Helen was able to acknowledge that, as much as the loss of her baby was a huge shock and reason for deep grief, she had quietly been preparing herself for such an outcome. Her instincts had been sending her messages about her fetus – instincts that she had listened to and then tried to subdue through rational thinking. Her story in this instance may not be a happy one, but it is a powerful illustration of the silent voice that lies within each of us.

Eleanor was at the hospital for a routine blood test and decided to pop into the antenatal clinic and request a midwife to listen in to her baby's heartbeat. She was not overly concerned but had noted a change in her baby's movements. The duty midwife soon found the baby's strong, regular heartbeat and she decided to measure Eleanor's abdomen. It came as a great shock to her when the midwife declared that Eleanor's baby was four weeks smaller than her dates suggested. An urgent ultrasound scan was arranged for the next day. Eleanor spent a very distressed evening; she had not been concerned about the size of her baby – this was, after all, her second pregnancy (and she was taller than average, 5ft 9in) – but had sought technology to confirm her belief that everything was well. Now there was some doubt. Luckily, the following day's scan proved she had been right – the baby was absolutely fine.

unborn children, and increased caution is a manifestation of this instinct. Thus instinct can change behaviour both in the short- and long term.

Throughout your pregnancy, as your baby develops in his safe sanctuary, his reassuring movements and patterns of behaviour – kicking, hiccupping, sleeping and waking – continue to tell you that all is well. Even at night, when you're asleep, your unconscious mind is registering every movement your baby makes. You will awaken instantly if you feel there is a problem; these instincts will surface immediately.

So, even when in utero, you and your partner know your baby better than anyone; you automatically have additional information that your healthcare professional does not. Moreover, you are the bearer of this child. The bond between him and you will be unique. Do not be afraid of using this bond to develop a better understanding of your baby, and make the right choices for him. Your instinct will become stronger day by day, and it will provide you with a formidable basis upon which to make decisions.

In her inspirational book, *Women's Bodies Women's Wisdom*, Dr. Christiane Northrup offers fascinating insights into female health and healing. She writes about how a woman's health is intrinsically linked to the culture in which

A doctor herself, Dr. Northrup says, "Each woman knows more about herself than anyone else."

she lives and her position therein, as well as the way in which a woman fulfils her life as an individual. She encourages women to "Awaken that still, small, intuitive voice in all of us, that voice of our own body that we have been forced to ignore through our culture's illness, misinformation and dysfunction." She describes the way many women are emotionally bound by cultural attitudes and what she terms the "addictive society". The beliefs that we subscribe to are limiting our ability to reclaim our female instinct, and empower ourselves. One example is how we have been socialized to consult with a medical professional whenever we are concerned about our health. The myth our society has created is that doctors know more than we do about our bodies.

How encouraging it would be to have an holistic relationship with your carer – be he or she a midwife, obstetrician or doctor – who also would help you to listen to your inner voice. Such a relationship also would encourage you to ask questions in a more open manner, and ultimately help you to acquire knowledge that might be uniquely associated with your situation. Equipped with factual information and increased awareness, supported in a sensitive way by your carer, you would start to hear the voice of your inner thoughts and have confidence in what they told you. As your instinctive awareness increased, you would become more effective at "monitoring" your baby around the clock, whether awake and "listening in" to your baby or subconsciously while you slept.

SIXTH SENSE

It often has been observed that human beings and animals who are born without one of their senses, or lose a sense during their lives, learn to rely more on their

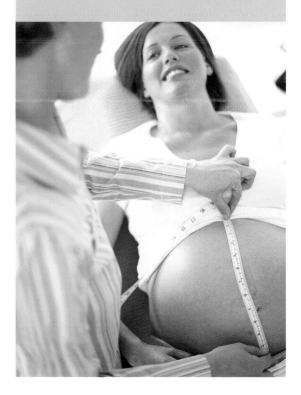

MEASURING THE FUNDUS

A common antenatal routine is to measure an expectant mother's abdomen to ensure a baby is growing in step with his gestational age. The measurement is assessed from the top of the bony symphysis pubis to the top of the uterus and involves calculating that one centimetre is equal to one week of pregnancy.

remaining senses, so that a sightless person may have acute hearing or greater kinaesthetic ability. This is also true of the sixth sense or our subconscious ability.

This phenomenon of heightened senses is active in pregnancy – especially during those early months, when your body is changing so fast you tend to be firing on all cylinders. Such heightened senses are particularly fortunate during the times when instinct is all that women have to "tell" them their babies are all right. Before a baby's movements are felt, we have to rely on our instincts to know that all is well and baby is healthy. First-time expectant mothers usually begin to feel the early movements of their unborn babies as "flutterings" between 20 and 25 weeks of pregnancy, and second-time expectant mothers some weeks sooner. Not only is this an incredible feeling, it also endorses your instinct that all is well with this new life.

Scanners and monitors identify only that you and your pregnancy are normal at the particular moments in time that they are used. So what happens the rest of the time?

Of course, in countries where scanning is available and used during early pregnancy, we are becoming less dependent on the use of instinct to monitor our babies. However, you need to realize that these procedures identify only that you and your pregnancy are normal at that particular moment in time. So what happens the rest of the time? Think about it. Yes, you will have to rely on your instincts. And what if you have cause for concern, to whom do you turn to seek reassurance? Do you deny your instincts in the hope that all is well, or will you be able to contact your midwife or healthcare practitioner knowing that she or he will empathize with your instinctive concerns?

REDISCOVERING YOUR INSTINCT

Instinct is very strong and powerful. It is deeply embedded in the mind and is active from a time before birth. Most of our primal instincts are written in our genes and form part of human survival – the need to hunt, protect and breed. Male and female instincts will differ, not only because each individual has a particular genetic make-up, but also due to the roles society affords the sexes. It is a biological fact that woman are the physical carriers of babies and that they are the providers of breast milk. Their biology, therefore, drives their instincts naturally to assume the nurturing role of parenthood.

We are born as strong and highly instinctive little beings. A newly born, full-term, baby has the most amazing ability to survive. Nature has provided him with a lusty cry that alerts his parents to the fact that something is conflicting with his needs – to be fed, watered, comforted – needs that are purely instinctive and driven by his developing brain. An infant also will have enough brown fat to sustain him for several days without food or water, and to some degree, ensure warmth. An amazing illustration of a baby's primal instinct to survive is, left unsupervised, a newborn placed on his mother's abdomen will move up towards her breast and attempt to feed.

Reflect for a moment on your instinctive development. At different times in your life you may feel that you have experienced different levels of instinct. As a newborn baby, your behaviour was driven by the instinct to survive and to maintain the continuum that began in the womb; you trusted that your mother had the ability to understand and respond. As a toddler, your environmental awareness became more selective. For example, when you were passed from your mother to another adult, you demonstrated your insecurity by crying out and reaching for the person who represented guaranteed security to you. As we mature and begin to develop the ability to reason, and process and understand facts, we add a new element of knowledge, one that tends to be more conscious, one that is cognitive and learned. This gradually becomes our minds' more automatic source of information, to the extent that we reduce our dependence on instinct and subconscious knowledge. In fact, at times, we may even use our brains to override our instincts. Yet there will be occasions when learned knowledge will not provide the answers to certain questions, so in those cases, our only option will be to seek answers further afield, or to look inward to our instinctive knowledge.

At no other time in a woman's life will those instincts be so important as during pregnancy and childbirth. You have instincts that will protect you and your baby throughout, but how can you begin to trust them if you are not fully aware of their existence? If you do acquire the ability to listen to your mind and body, they will serve you in good stead. Not only will you feel that you have more control over what is happening to you during pregnancy and birth, but you may also begin to feel a closer connection with your baby.

There are so many ways we can get to know our bodies and the messages they transmit. It may seem intangible and somewhat of an enigma yet, without exception, we all have the ability to tune in to our "inner knowing". The actual means that you use to understand your body is not important, but over time, hopefully you will develop the ability to concentrate your mind on understanding the thoughts and messages coming from within. In essence, getting in touch with the inner you is about switching off the routines and expectations of the immediate and everyday world and crossing from the tangible and conscious to a more intuitive and subconscious state. You may not need to do this in a structured class-led environment such as yoga or group meditation. Simply sitting down in a quiet space and taking the time to reflect will expose many channels of which you may be unaware.

Dr. Northrup believes that by listening to your own body and by trusting in its wisdom, a healing journey will begin that will induce physical and spiritual wellness. She says: "Central to this vision is that we trust what we know in our bones: that our bodies are our allies and that they will always point us in the direction we need to go next." She talks of our intuitive capacity that needs to be re-accessed, through greater use of the intelligence that lies within each of us but is rarely accessed during everyday life. She advocates tapping in to this knowledge and acting accordingly, in tandem with a re-evaluation of what our emotions are telling us, in spite of the status quo laid down by the culture and society within which we live. She says: "When we realign with our inner guidance and stop judging our bodies and our feelings as bad when they are offering us information, we are on the pathway to a life filled with growth and delight."

GETTING IN TOUCH WITH YOUR BABY

Communicating with your baby will take place at both a conscious and subconscious level. By the time your baby is kicking regularly and, even more, when his birth is impending, you will probably find it quite natural to talk to your baby, and maybe even sing to him. However, in the early days, when your baby is only a fraction of an inch long, it may seem strange to talk away and communicate with him. Yet rest assured – this is when subconscious communication first occurs.

There are many ways of communicating: you can speak or sing to your baby; play music or other sounds; or use your mental and/or spiritual powers.

Just by placing your hand on your tummy, as I have seen so many pregnant women do in the most instinctive and unaware fashion, you are telling your baby that you know he is there, you are thinking about him, and that you are protecting him and keeping him safe.

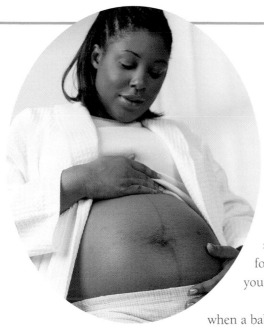

You are a "mother" to your baby well before he is born. During the nine months of pregnancy you are providing all the nurturing care that you can and he will arrive expecting you to continue to safeguard his wellbeing.

Some methods are more obvious than others but they are all effective in their own way, and will help you and your baby to start bonding. Don't worry about finding a form of communication that feels natural for you and your baby, you will.

There are many different theories as to when a baby is able to distinguish sounds from his outside environment, and how he may respond to these sounds. Dr. Thomas Verny writes in detail about the experience he believes a baby encounters during his time in utero. In his book, *The Secret Life of the Unborn Child*, Verny quotes studies that show how the unborn child has the ability to hear from the 24th week onwards, allowing him to listen to voices and sounds from outside the protected environment of the womb. Verny provides many anecdotes of circumstantial evidence as to the way in which an unborn child tunes into his external environment and how this may influence his postnatal reactions.

Dr. Verny also believes that it is possible to begin teaching an unborn baby to respond to what it feels and hears, simply by listening to relaxing music for a few minutes each day. Music is a very tangible and expressive way of communicating with your unborn child, and depending on the type of music selected, it can have a stimulating or calming effect on both you and your baby. It is not uncommon for a mother to wonder at how her young baby calms down as soon as he hears a particular track of music – one that was played frequently during her pregnancy. Women who practice yoga, relaxation, or just have a quiet bath with music playing in the background, often find this effect particularly profound, as they have started an association in the womb between specific music and a peaceful moment of calm. In fact, this is one way of helping the transition from a baby's in utero existence to his life outside the womb. Babies love to feel safe and be surrounded by touch, smells and sounds that are familiar. The interaction between their instincts and senses and the outside world provides them with a continuum from the womb. The more familiar this interaction is with that experienced inside the womb, the more will be their acceptance of their outside existence.

SINGING AND TALKING

Singing is another form of music that can be used to activate the communication process before a baby is born. Maybe you sing to an older child before sleep, or maybe you start singing the same song to your unborn baby before you sleep at night. So much of a child's first year is about association, and the relationship that it develops between singing and relaxation can be very calming for the newborn. Many people who do not feel comfortable talking to their unborn children find that singing is a more natural source of communication. A song can be about anything; it doesn't have to be a love song or a lullaby! Just to be able to sing a set of words in a melody will create that initial recognition that provides the link between a baby's pre- and postnatal existence. Singing is also a wonderful way for an older child to communicate with a younger brother or sister. Thus the bond between siblings can commence right there in the womb.

For those who are able to talk to their unborn children, this is a lovely form of communication. Talking to your belly may seem like a strange idea, yet if your baby can hear your voice and makes an association between it and someone who provides comfort in the outside world, this sheds a different light on the prospect. You realize you are not talking to a belly, you are talking to a human being who can understand and probably even interact with you from within the womb. You, too, are starting to bond with your baby before it is born.

Many couples give their unborn baby a name or term of endearment, bringing them closer to this little person as an individual. This may not be the eventual name of the child, in fact it may not be a name at all! But it is your way of addressing this little being who is part of your physical body. It is a way of starting to refer to this being as a member of the family, and this verbal communication will undoubtedly reinforce your baby's emotional wellbeing as he is reminded on a regular basis of his place in the family.

UNSPOKEN COMMUNICATION

Not all communication is verbal, however. Silent communication is often the most powerful type, as it engages the mind in a different way. It involves thoughts, emotions and feelings. Again, Dr. Verny discusses how a baby can pick up on the emotions and feelings of his mother, in a way that paves his perception of life, expectations and even certain behaviours. The sensitive bond between mother and child is so strong that your two bodies together can form a channel of communication without the need for spoken dialogue. Elisabeth Hallett describes some amazing experiences of pre-birth communication in her book, *Stories of the Unborn Soul*. Many of the stories recounted are a result of meditation, although this is not always the case. She offers stunning insights into the ability of an unborn child to reach his parents and, if necessary, to guide them through the process of pregnancy and birth.

Dreaming is another expression of our inner knowing and is also a useful outlet for unresolved emotions, fears and possible ambivalence. In his book, *The Dreaming Mind*, Robert Van der Castle discusses the way in which we dream during pregnancy and some of the symbolism associated with these dreams. He describes how women have dreamed of meeting their babies before they are born, and of how real the vision of the dream was once the baby was born. He believes that this is also a start to the bonding process, as a relationship between parent and child starts in dreams and quiet moments of reflection. As a pregnancy advances towards birth, the wonderfully instinctive partnership between mother and baby progresses harmoniously towards the ultimate in communication between two minds and two bodies – the birth.

Bear in mind that your baby is preparing himself for being born just as you are preparing yourself for his arrival.

Massage is another powerful form of nonverbal communication. The benefits of massage are becoming more widely accepted in Western society, and when better to start massaging your baby than in the womb. Establishing this kind of hand-to-body contact with your baby while he is in utero will create another familiar feeling to which your baby will respond. In fact, you may feel him physically change position in order to come toward the surface of your abdomen and to feel the movements of your hands.

As I have said before, there are many ways of communicating, and you will find whichever suits you best. Communication is very powerful and will be of benefit to all parties involved. The birth of a baby is as challenging and exciting an event for him, as it is for you and your partner. In fact, a vaginal birth probably requires a baby to do more than 50 percent of the work! As your baby leaves the sanctuary of your womb towards the unknown territory of his new world, he will be looking for every piece of reassurance and familiarity he can find. Your voice and presence will be a great source of comfort to your new baby; the sooner you get close to your baby, the better his happy continuum will be preserved.

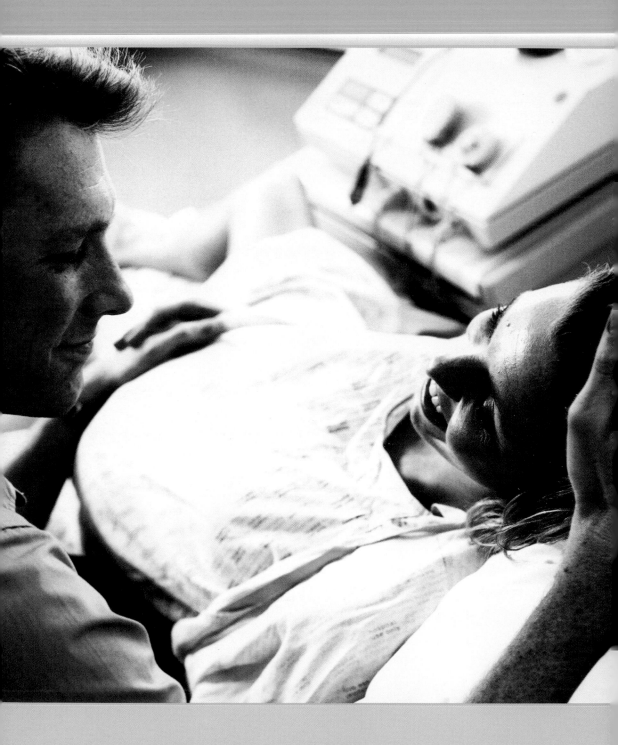

CHAPTER 6
Preparing for Birth

✳ PREPARING FOR BIRTH

The idea of having a baby can be a very romantic and exciting thought. From the moment a pregnancy test is positive, visions of baby clothes, cots, prams and cuddly toys spring to mind. Every time we turn on the television, there are smiling tots running around in their nappies to greet us; their chubby legs, round faces and adorable smiles reinforcing our idea of cute. Planning for this adorable little being, what he is going to be called, and how he is going to look can consume literally hours and hours of any couple's time. Those first few months of pregnancy are so full of questions, ideas and dreams for the future. Then, all too quickly, 36 weeks have passed and everything that has been discussed and dreamed of is about to become reality.

The final days arrive and with them come a new set of thoughts and concerns that, up until now, may have been bubbling beneath the surface. The nesting instinct, that urge to have all things neat and tidy and everything on hand, may manifest as the ultimate stages of preparation are completed. The planning, and possibly dry run, of the journey to the hospital needs to be reviewed. The hospital bag, with all the right things, has to be packed. If this baby is not your first, you'll need to arrange the care of your other children. The experience of labour may now seem uncomfortably close and, of course, there's the very real prospect of actually becoming a parent.

Some couples approach the final days of pregnancy with a feeling of challenging anticipation and excitement. Others may panic as they begin to take on board the reality of the impending events.

DUE DATES

One of the first potential hurdles to overcome is the notion of a "due date". Term can fall anywhere between 37 and 43 weeks, so there is genuine ambiguity around the notion of the expected date of delivery. I often wish that mothers could be provided with a timescale and a probability date, but not an exact date towards which they and, more importantly, "the system", work. This would help with the psychology of dealing with the last days. It also would bode well emotionally for the soon-to-be parents, as they would no longer be tied to one date that causes frustration, impatience and growing concern as soon as it passes and the possibility of induction of labour arises.

A degree of frustration may well start to emerge when a mother has gone beyond this magical date she has been given and starts saying things like "Come on baby, don't be lazy, time to get a move on!" Or "This baby has kicked me so much, it is so naughty." I always feel so defensive for that little baby when I hear such comments, as the baby doesn't know how to be lazy and it certainly does not know how to be naughty! And he may be feeling squeezed into a space that he is fast outgrowing.

It is nature that decrees when the birthing process is ready to begin. We know some, but by no means all, of the hormonal activity between mother and baby

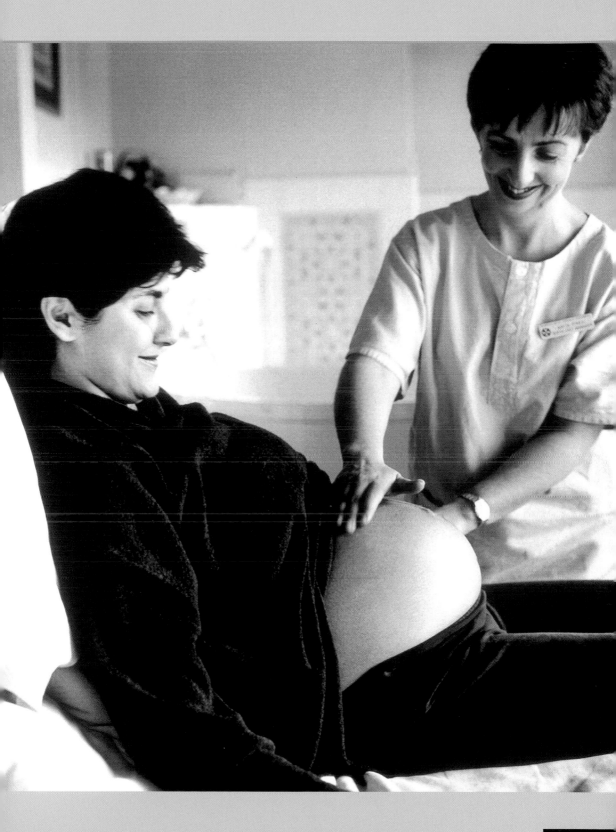

responsible for triggering labour. Of course, all the frustration demonstrated by a mother is natural, considering how long she has waited to hold her baby in her arms. But nature has the last word and this baby will arrive when he is ready.

It is interesting that different cultures measure the duration of pregnancy in different ways. For example, in the East, they tend to follow the lunar calendar, estimating term based on the passing of ten full lunar cycles. This can fall anywhere between 280 and 307 days, during which time minimal levels of intervention are practiced. We know that anxiety inhibits not only the onset but also the progress of labour, yet in the West, we continue to burden mothers with this unnecessary pressure.

IMAGINING PARENTHOOD

Another challenge to overcome during those final weeks is the notion of impending parenthood. There are those expectant parents who tend to think the ideal scenario is one in which a baby sleeps, feeds and has his nappy changed with a little play now and again. Then there are those who have been scared by the media, and even their friends, into thinking that all their baby is going to do is to keep them up all night and cry and feed all day long. Having only ever been a spectator to other new parents, a couple's idea of

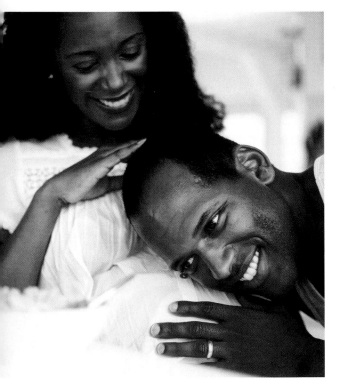

parenthood is a result of all the images, examples and experiences they may have had, to date none of which are their own. As they reach the final weeks of pregnancy, most mothers have started to reflect on what sort of parent they hope to be, based on their experiences, their beliefs, and their observations of others. They also try to imagine what the partnership of parenthood is going to be like for themselves and their partners, as the two of them embark on this new chapter in their lives.

With the birth approaching, a couple may be exploring their feelings, those they have for each other and those they will have as a family. Some mothers-to-be are almost consumed with love for this new little being from the moment of conception. For others, mother love only begins to grow once the baby is safely there. There is no rule book. Reality will probably be very different from what you have imagined. As much as we may envisage and identify the skills we may bring to our new role as a parent, the reality is often quite different. In fact, one of the common post-birth challenges experienced by new parents is the process of readjusting many of the expectations that they had built up during their pregnancies.

As you approach your due date, you will benefit by thinking about the positive aspects of what lies ahead. This is a good time to seek out favourable attitudes wherever possible. Anticipate the wonderful moment when you will be holding your baby in your arms for the first time, think about the intimacies of breastfeeding, and imagine creating a unique bond with your baby. All soon-to-be-mothers should be encouraged to listen to their innermost feelings and to commune with their babies, rather than fixating on the prospect of sleepless nights, overwhelming emotions, and the times when their babies may be crying for no obvious reason. In the majority of cases, the doubts of parenthood soon subside and life settles down into some sort of a pattern, especially if the extended family is on hand.

A baby does not have to change everything, but having the time to spend with your child is something you will rarely regret, so taking the time to think about how this can be achieved is time well spent.

TIME CONSTRAINTS

Many of today's mothers, however, lack the needed time to prepare themselves physically and mentally for the impending change. A lot of women work and are still in the "job comes first" mindset. In terms of personal preparation, many women are not able to allow themselves to feel special, to care for themselves, or to be nurtured as they approach these final days of pregnancy. Throughout this book I have stressed how important it is that an expectant mother re-evaluates where she is in her life, and that she must prioritize what she's looking for.

Time being of the essence applies to those weeks prior to birth as much as to the ensuing months. While it is physically possible to work until the birth of your baby or a week before, have a great birth, and settle into motherhood quite successfully, the signs of over-exertion will inevitably show at some point. You need time before the birth of your child to gather yourself, both mentally and physically. You may have to relinquish some of your pre-baby life and associated responsibilities, in order to open up space into which your baby can fit. It is very easy to think of the physical space that a baby requires, but the mental and emotional aspects are less tangible. Therefore, it is important to have in place a solid foundation of mental and psychological strength along with the physical ability to cope. Some countries are very good at recognizing this need, and have legislation in place that allows a woman to leave work a few weeks prior to birth without it jeopardizing her financial commitments. And, in a few countries, it is mandatory to leave work at least a few weeks prior to the birth of a baby and the expecting mother is strongly encouraged to rest.

Unfortunately not all countries are as evolved in the way they approach maternity care and provision of maternity pay. Where the maternity policies are less favourable, women are often obliged to work through the entirety of their pregnancies. For them, it is quite a challenge to get into the mindset I described. Although there is often a choice as to when to take paid maternity leave, many women want to take the majority of the time after their babies arrive, which is understandable. For these women, working until 38 or 39 weeks seems sensible, not only for financial reasons, but sometimes just because they enjoy being busy and feel that the challenge of work may reduce the feeling of endless waiting at the end. But they may also find it more difficult to take a step back from the buzz of everyday life and contemplate some of the changes about to take place, especially if work consumes a high level of mental and physical energy. Because of the role that is enforced upon women these days, and the joint financial burden they often share with their partners, many will maximize their paid maternity during the postnatal period, even if it means they overexert themselves towards the latter end of their pregnancy.

Once a woman has decided to have a baby, be it planned or unplanned, both she and her partner need to rethink their aspirations and possibly even reset their expectations.

Generally, there seems to be a global consensus that the first six to twelve months post birth is a very important time for a mother and baby. As a consequence, even if a woman is not paid for the entire duration, she should be allowed to stay at home and return to the same job thereafter. While some progress has been made towards achieving this goal, there is still an outstanding financial requirement that has not been fully addressed by many countries.

Governments should be encouraging enterprise to take a more family-friendly approach to the work environment. Most companies still struggle with the reality of flexible working, both for males and females. Yet the onus cannot be placed entirely on the government and employers. We as individuals need to make some of the changes. We should reset our expectations, by opening ourselves up to a wider support network, and by working with employers to help them to support the family environment. Change is good and society would not progress without it.

Yet sometimes we need to take a step back from constant progress and completely reassess our values and basic needs. In my quest to have women heed their instincts, I accept that a balance between what nature intended and what our current mindset allows has to be struck. Living in the 21st century, it is not feasible to expect women who have progressed so far to revert to the old days where a career and financial responsibility lay exclusively in the male domain. But it would be nice to imagine that, while planning for a new baby, a couple starts to envisage the possibility of the mother giving up work several weeks before term and spending six months to a year at home after the birth. It is interesting that many women who have babies and the intention of resuming work quite soon afterwards, actually decide not to return once they have their babies in their arms. Their financial contribution becomes less important, or they are able to find ways of working around the situation. But that is when the strong emotional bond has kicked in; it is not the same before a baby is born. Ideally, we need to consider how to convince a couple before their baby is born that their child will revolutionize their outlook on life, including their views of their financial status.

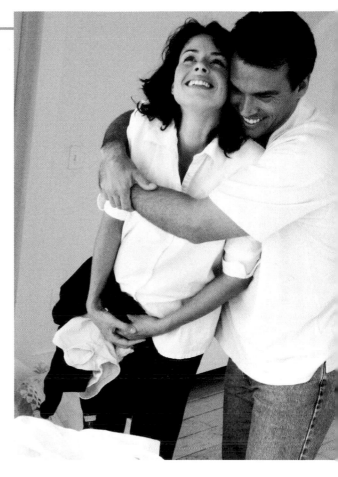

The final days of pregnancy can be both exciting and trepidatious. There's all the fun of imagining the expected arrival and making the necessary preparations but there also are worries about what the birth will be like.

What often puts a couple's financial priorities into a new perspective is an inability to conceive a child. Couples who are desperate for a baby will often spend a small fortune, finding the will and the way to obtain funding to have that longed-for baby. When it comes to creating and giving birth to a baby, there always seems to be a pot of money that can be found, in order that the dream materializes. Yet once the baby has arrived, there seems to be less commitment to finding those extra pennies that allow a mother and child to spend quality time together.

GETTING ACQUAINTED WITH THE BIRTH ENVIRONMENT

Preparation for the physical birth itself can be an exciting activity, and one that can be shared with your partner. As an expectant mother, you should be provided with the opportunity to familiarize yourself with your birthing environment, even if this is a provisional decision. If you plan on having your baby in hospital, it is very useful for you to become accustomed to the terminology and appearance of the equipment that may be employed during the birth. In order for your tour to be fully informative, it should be conducted by a qualified midwife who is fully capable of describing the hospital's protocols and policies, and who will be able to explain the appropriate use of technology and equipment. On such a tour, a midwife can present the pros and cons of what she is demonstrating in a relaxed manner, and you'll be stimulated to pose questions that you might not ask in a less visible setting. The reality of the situation may further influence your decision-making to the extent that you may be prompted to explore alternatives.

*   Annette, a 40-year-old mother expecting her sixth baby, let me know during my consultation visit that she didn't wish to have any pregnancy tests whatsoever. She was a highly intelligent and well-informed woman, and had decided after the birth of her first child not to submit to routine pregnancy testing. She had documented evidence of her blood group and rhesus factor. Refreshingly, she totally trusted her very strong instincts – acquired during her five previously healthy pregnancies. She did not wish her unborn baby to be disturbed. She even requested that I not use the sonicaid, which amplifies the fetal hearbeat, but instead use the Pinnard's stethoscope (an old-fashioned trumpet-like instrument, which is placed on the mother's abdomen and picks up the heartbeat after about 28 weeks' pregnancy). I was very happy to oblige this determined mother. The labour and birth, which took place at home, was completely straightforward and I felt justified in never questioning the integrity of this wise and experienced woman. Some mothers have complained to me that they've been told they are selfish and not thinking of their babies when they attempt to follow their instincts. In my experience, nothing could be further from the truth.

FETAL POSITIONING

This is another aspect of pre-birth preparation that may have an impact on your birthing experience. As you approach term, hopefully you will know that your baby is not only in the head-down position, but also that his back is facing towards the front of your abdomen, in the "anterior" position. This information will be discussed between you and your midwife or obstetrician, who has been able to use her experience to locate your baby's head and track its progress into your pelvis. Should your baby not be lying in the optimum fetal position, you will be advised about positions you can adopt in order to encourage your unborn baby to assume the ideal position for labour and birth. There are many suggested techniques for turning a baby into the optimum position, such as crawling on all fours, swimming and rocking on a birthing ball. Many complementary therapists also claim success in turning a baby, especially from a breech or posterior position, so there are several alternatives available. As with many aspects of pregnancy and birth, some level of control is retained by the baby and, of course, by nature. Consequently, part of the pre-birth preparation may be to accept the position that your baby has adopted, and consider how you may want to adapt your plans accordingly, bearing in mind that a baby may change his position during labour. Many mothers whose babies have not progressed into the ideal position prior to the onset of labour are still able to labour and birth them naturally, but others may choose to have a caesarean.

LIE OF THE BABY

The best position for your baby to adopt is occiput anterior: head down with his back facing your abdomen. If his back is turned towards your spine, this is occiput posterior, which can cause severe backache in labour. About 4 percent of babies settle bottom or feet first, known as breech presentation. Less than 1 percent of babies are positioned across the uterus, which is known as transverse lie. Breech presentation may result in a cesarean delivery, while a transverse lie definitely will. Ultimately, it is the baby whose head has descended into the pelvis before labour (head is engaged), whose back is lying to the front of his mother's abdomen (ideally to the left) for whom labour and birth should be the most straight-forward. The further down the birth canal the baby has progressed before labour, the shorter labour will be. Conversely if the baby's head is high in the birth canal or he is lying in the "posterior" position (with his back facing towards the mother's back), labour may be longer. An expectant mother whose baby is in the posterior position should be prepared that her labour, especially the latent and first stage, will take considerably longer, and that she should be afforded unlimited time in which to labour and birth. Of course, there will be exceptions.

> ✳ I recall a 40-year-old first-time mother who was labouring beautifully in a birthing pool and making excellent progress. Suddenly, she began to spontaneously birth her baby. To our utter amazement, her 8-lb son arrived gazing upwards in the direct posterior position after a labour of just seven hours from beginning to end!

ANTENATAL CLASSES

Another useful and very tangible form of pre-birth preparation is to attend antenatal sessions; you can learn a great deal and have the opportunity for questions and discussion. They vary in content and delivery style, so it is worth understanding what the focus of any class will be. Many women enjoy the topics covered, as well as the fact that others may ask questions they did not feel comfortable asking.

I encourage couples to structure their sessions to suit their individual needs. The first session is spent brainstorming in order to prioritize what they hope to obtain from subsequent sessions, giving the participants the opportunity to be in control of the content and using me as a source of relevant information. I am also acutely aware that fathers-to-be very often have their own agendas and that it is important to provide them with a safe forum within which they can ask and receive experiential knowledge, equipping them in their role as birth supporter. I usually close sessions with a group discussion, so that any other topics, questions and concerns can be discussed together.

Another useful aspect of antenatal classes is being able to hear from other mothers who come along to recount their recent birthing tales. I am always very selective as to the women I invite. I naturally call upon women who have had wonderful birth experiences, so we can see their joy and, thus, reinforce our own aspirations. I also ask women who feel that they could have done things slightly differently, so that the mothers-to-be can learn from them and their experiences.

Finally antenatal classes provide an opportunity to meet other expectant couples, and to share your thoughts, concerns and expectations with them. Many friendships blossom and sometimes continue long after the babies have arrived. In the absence of a close support network and family, these friendships can become your lifeline. It is so easy to believe that you are the only one going through the challenges presented by pregnancy, so having the opportunity to share these with other couples who may well have encountered similar experiences, is invaluable. What, in fact, you are achieving in these friendships is developing your own support group of like-minded people.

LEVEL OF PREPARATION

Different people like to prepare for a big event in different ways. Some like to have everything in "ship-shape" order before the big day, safe in the knowledge that they have catered for most eventualities. Some like to "wing" it; arrive on the day and go with the flow. Birth is no exception and it's important to acknowledge that either can be just as effective. Planners have probably spent more time reading, thinking, and mulling over some of the "what if" scenarios that may occur. They probably also have detailed birth plans that summarize their aspirations. Such women are more likely to be in control. That said, they also are more likely to be disappointed if their actual experience is not as they had planned. Those women who arrive on the scene with little or no preparation have probably given much less thought to the event. They may encounter some surprises along the route, but they are much less likely to be disappointed, as they did not arrive with many preconceived ideas.

Of course there is a happy medium and that is to seek out information, have the ability to make informed choices but, wherever possible, to keep an open mind. This way you have an understanding of what is happening and why. You will have a tendency to panic less and will probably retain a level of control in any decisions taken, thus increasing your chance of making the best decision based on your specific circumstances. This will stand you in good stead for the next 20 years!

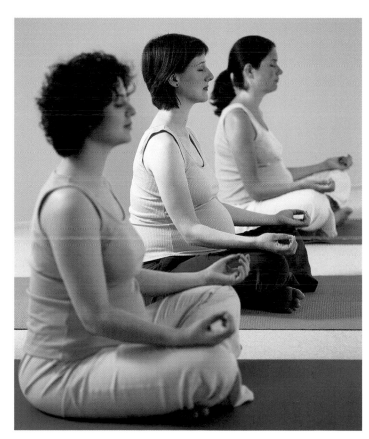

There are many different options available in antenatal classes, depending on your beliefs, birth aspirations and their requirements. Many teach meditation as a way of relaxing the mind and body before birth.

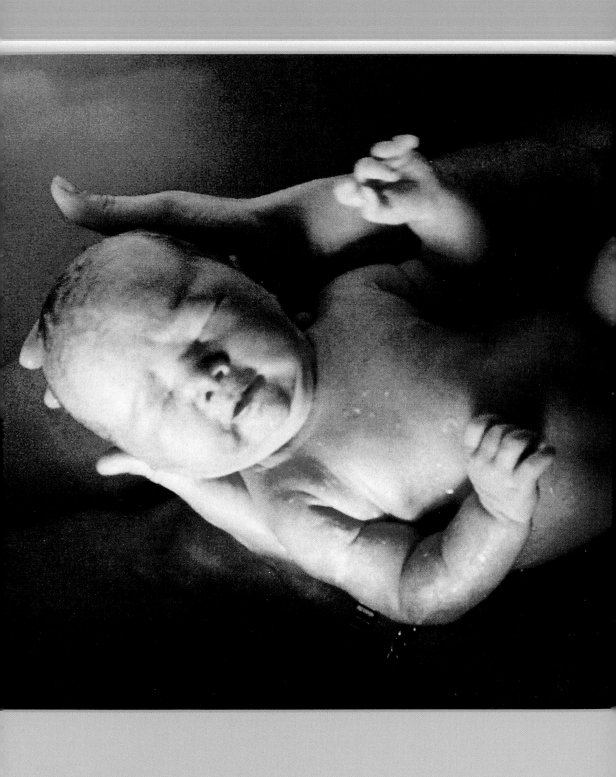

CHAPTER 7
Instinctive Birthing

✳ INSTINCTIVE BIRTHING

In many ways, this is the most important chapter of the book; words, thoughts and opinions so far expressed come together for this incredible event – the birth. I recall with mixed feelings the birth of my own four boys, all of whom were induced. I succumbed to the routine practice of the time, and was ignorant of the things I've experienced since working as a midwife.

More vivid are the memories I carry from the many births I have been privileged to attend during my long professional career; each one represents a very unique memory. Birthing a baby is one of the most intimate events of human life. At the very least, two people are involved, mother and baby. The way in which these two individuals communicate, interact and work together is an essential part of the birth experience. As your pregnancy advances towards term, you and those around you will tend to concentrate very much on the physical nature of the forthcoming birth, but this is only part of the overall picture. Beneath the surface lies a bubbling sea of hormonal, emotional and metaphysical influences that may play a significant role in the final outcome. As with all the intangible and unexplained aspects of life, our society often pretends to understand such influences but then acts in a way that suggests otherwise.

One of the joys of being a midwife is to believe in a woman's ability to tune in to those invisible factors, and to provide the individualized and appropriate support at all levels to a labouring woman. Naturally, if a relationship has been formed between a woman and her midwife prior to the birth, this level of understanding will be easier to attain than if you meet for the first time in the labour ward.

I believe a woman's first birthing experience is one of the most profound and far-reaching events of her life. At the very least, her first labour experience will undoubtedly influence her perception of subsequent pregnancies, labours and births. This chapter reflects birth as I have witnessed it. As you read the chapter, I hope you will begin to understand the way in which nature intended birth. In essence, this will be your body and mind left alone to intertwine and work freely to empower your instincts to influence the final outcome.

Traditionally the midwife is not merely a birth attendant with special expertise. She has a spiritual function in helping the baby to birth, the woman to become a mother, and in creating the setting for birth and the time immediately following it so that it is right for this spiritual transition. In many birth cultures she is responsible for prayers, chants, invocations, and other actions to clear the way for birth and to nurture the right relationships between all those participating.

Sheila Kitzinger *Rediscovering Birth*

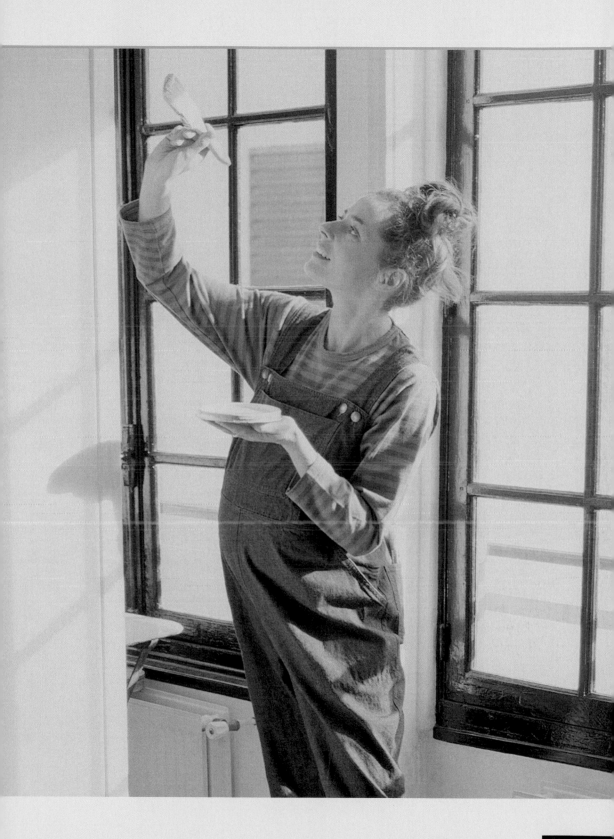

DIFFERENT WAYS OF BIRTHING

There still are cultures in the world where birth is considered a sacred activity belonging solely to women. Male partners are excluded from births and, if there are attendants or loved ones available to assist, they are other women. In Western society, birthing attendants will vary according to the location of birth, the progress of the labour and the nature of the birth. In the UK, if you decide to birth at home with non-invasive pain relief, you will be assisted by one dedicated midwife and one support midwife, available at all times. Unless there is an unforeseen complication, it is unlikely you would be seen by an obstetrician.

If, however, you elect to birth your baby in the hospital, you may be attended by one or more unfamiliar midwives, depending on the timing of the birth in relation to any shift rota changes. If you request an epidural, an anaesthetist also will need to be in attendance. In recent times, our approach to birth has involved much more activity and external influences. First-time mothers are all too often unaware of this, and therefore do not proactively seek to explore all the possibilities before submitting themselves to the prevailing routine.

In *Birth Reborn*, Michel Odent talks about the natural inclination a woman will show towards birthing privately if given the opportunity to be instinctive. He refers to a subconscious state that a woman will often reach during labour. This is a primal state of mind that a woman can find when she is at her most instinctive.

Two of "my" recent mothers experienced two very different situations, which illustrate the power of the sub-conscious mind. One was immersed safely in the warm water of her birthing pool almost ready to birth her third baby. She related that with each powerful contraction she felt as if she was dancing! The other, however, about to birth her second child at home, suddenly lunged towards me announcing with what appeared to be total conviction, that she felt as though she was going to die! Reaching for her pulse I quickly reassured her this was not the case.

The role of the midwife or birth attendant should be one of silent partner, supporting the woman and her baby through a profoundly intuitive birthing experience. I feel incredibly privileged to have witnessed an untold number of totally intuitive births. Many have been achieved in a hospital labour room with more than a degree of difficulty, and my colleagues always respected the fact that unless invited in for a specific reason, my ethos of care allowed a woman to find her own "place" while in labour.

CREATING THE ENVIRONMENT FOR INSTINCTIVE BIRTHING

The atmosphere that surrounds a mother is extremely important; even a mother whose pregnancy and birth is influenced by medical or obstetric complications has the right to be supported with complete sensitivity. If pregnancy and labour remain uncomplicated, caregivers should not create complications. The more comfortable, familiar and relaxed the environment, the more a woman will feel at ease and in control. This does not mean that you have to deliver at home to experience this kind of birth. There is no reason why you should not birth your baby safely and without intervention in the hospital, if that is the environment within which you feel safest. If you labour well and use your body to cope with the pain, you will be supported as much or as little as you need by the midwives.

Focus your mind on yourself and your baby. Your birthing partner and caregivers are there to offer you quiet encouragement and to help you feel safe and able to connect with your instinctive self.

It's especially important that when in labour, you free yourself from any extraneous thoughts and remain focused on yourself and your baby. Other participants should not talk or try to disturb you. This may be difficult for your birthing partner, particularly if he or she has not experienced childbirth before. Your birth partner may not be able to empathize and react accordingly, particularly when you reach further into your inner state of subconsciousness. It's important that you prepare your birthing partner for this possibility. He or she should be encouraged to see this quiet presence as an essential part of instinctive childbirth and to understand that mute reassurance can be of great support to you while labouring and may, in fact, be all you require. Midwives, too, can become fazed by a mother's singularly individual displays of instinctive behaviour, especially during the advanced stages of labour.

We approach birth quite differently from that of our mammalian counterparts. Female mammals, ready to give birth, will seek safe and private places, sanctuaries where they will birth their young on their own. They are likely to choose dimly lit, secure areas, away from potential predators and interference. They will spend the first few hours with their young, away from the danger and activity of the external world. They instinctively know that interruption will delay or stop the process of labour, and it won't resume until they feel at ease to continue.

By appreciating the patterns of animals and their need for quiet and safe labour environments, we can begin to get closer to instinctive human behaviour. Nature is infallibly protective of the perpetuation of the species. Just as females in the animal kingdom will respond adversely to external influences, so, too, will a labouring woman who is distracted by noise, environmental disturbances, unnecessary interventions and the presence of many strangers. If distracted, a woman will often revert to a "safe" mode, in which labour is prolonged while she accustoms herself to her changing environment. A well-documented example of this phenomenon is the diminution of contractions that may result when a mother in established labour transfers from one location to another. So finely tuned are the hormones of labour, of which we actually know very little but are discovering more all the time, that any disturbance in their balance will have a major effect on a labouring woman. Time will be needed before her body and mind become accustomed to the change in her environment. Such disturbances also prevent a mother from being in touch with her instincts, her body and her baby.

In recognition of the importance of seclusion and security in childbirth, more midwifery-led, low-tech, no-tech, birth centres are appearing. A reflection of their importance and a desire by many mothers to use such facilities is the fact that most, if not all, are over-subscribed. Midwives, too, are benefiting. They are accumulating experience of a holistic hands-on approach, and living up to their title of midwife, which means literally "with woman". From a midwife's perspective, an instinctive birth is all about being there for a woman, empowering her to be in control. Such a presence enables a woman to feel safe, and maximizes her instinctive response to the demands that nature will normally present in order for labour to progress.

Mothers have to work incredibly hard to labour and to birth their babies in a way that honours their instinctive and primal needs. A sensitive midwife will be cognizant of this, and will encourage a mother to identify and listen to her inner feelings, releasing her inhibitions to voice those messages, and to work alongside them. Mothers deprived of sensitive caring and experienced support and reassurance throughout their pregnancies are often, at the very least, apprehensive, and at worst, scared of childbirth, disbelieving that nature has prepared their bodies and their babies for this momentous life event. We know for a fact that fear intensifies pain. How wrong is it then that we deprive so many mothers, especially first-time mothers, of their innate ability to welcome the truly amazing experience that lies before them.

Apprehension is natural and in many ways healthy. A woman about to give birth should not be enclosed in a cocoon of fear, but should be able to express her worries and concerns to her midwife, who will help her to transform those feelings into excitement and anticipation. This should be a time when a pregnant woman's instincts, coupled with her accumulated knowledge, and supported by her known and trusted carers, will facilitate her mind and body to react constructively and spontaneously as her labour begins.

THE ROLE OF FATHERS-TO-BE

At a recent consultation I was asked what I perceived to be the role of the father-to-be during childbirth. My view is, and always has been, that the role of the father has to be whatever the woman in labour desires. However, if you're having your first baby, you will probably not be able to foretell exactly what your needs and feelings will be. Therefore, it is vitally important that the expectant father is aware of this possibility, and that he is prepared for the fact that you may well behave completely out of character. Of

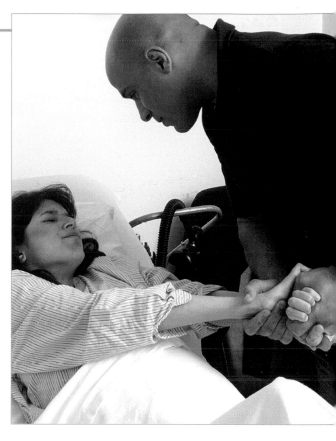

In the West, differently to more traditional cultures, women often rely on their partners to be present at their births, to comfort and sustain them, and to share in the experience of bringing their children into the world.

Jane, a first-time mother, remonstrated quite forcefully when anyone touched her once her contractions began. She instinctively wanted only to pace to and fro, vigorously massaging her own back until the contraction subsided. She was in total control of what her body required, and her partner was reassured that simply by being present, he was helping and supporting her, even though he felt superfluous to her needs.

course, you, too, should prepare yourself for this possibility! For example, you may swear and vocalize with increasing frequency and volume as your labour advances. This can be extremely off-putting and even distressing for a first-time father-to-be.

The way in which a woman desires physical and mental support during active labour is very individual. What may appear to a birthing partner to be changeable emotions and demands are actually the responses of a woman totally in concert with the ways her body wants to manage the contractions. Wanting to be touched one minute and then not at all the next may seem irrational but, trust me, it is perfectly normal! One of the most important aspects of being a birthing partner is to respect these needs and accept that your role may be passive or active, but whatever the case, your responding "correctly" to your partner is what matters.

MANAGING WITHOUT A BIRTH PARTNER

So what of the husband or partner who would really prefer not to attend the labour or birth? Or a woman who, for her own reasons, prefers that her partner does not attend? She should not feel that she has to succumb to pressure to do otherwise, as this mother is following an instinct that is protecting her from unnecessary pressure at her most vulnerable moment. Should a woman choose to labour alone or with another individual at her side, this decision needs to be understood and respected, even if it is contrary to the status quo and the expectations set down by modern-day society. The midwife can and should encourage dialogue between a couple to ensure both partners have the

* I remember when Sally called me to her first labour. Upon my arrival at her home she was surrounded by loving friends and relatives, who were unintentionally making it almost impossible for me to observe the extent of her progress. Not wishing to appear obtrusive I remained passively in the background until it became obvious that Sally was struggling and unable to succumb fully to her labouring body due to the cacophony of noise surrounding her. I respectfully suggested to Sally that maybe she would labour more efficiently if the room was quieter. She agreed and asked the guests to leave. She then advanced quite rapidly in her labour and successfully birthed her baby son in the birthing pool.

opportunity to explore their individual feelings and needs surrounding this incredibly important life event. A sensitive and intuitive midwife can often detect when a husband or partner is struggling with the sight of his loved one in advanced labour, and can facilitate the opportunity for him to "take some air", reassuring him that all is well with mother and unborn baby. Occasionally, a husband, partner, the woman's mother, or indeed any relative can inhibit labour's progress. Again, sensitivity on the part of the midwife is the order of the day. Should she perceive that labour is being impeded, she should suggest a subtle alternative.

There are some women, particularly those expecting a baby for the first time, who in making preparations for their births, believe that the experience will be enhanced by being surrounded by carefully chosen birth attendants. This may well be the case, but equally, once birthing, a woman may find herself in conflict with her pre-birth beliefs. It's very important, particularly in the case of a mother who has intricately planned her labour and birth and communicated her wishes to all those around her, that should she change her mind at any time, she should not be made to feel embarrassed or guilty.

LABOUR AS NATURE INTENDED

Both you and your baby are about to embark on a journey, a journey of a lifetime. Labour is an experience about which we know so much and, ironically, about which we also know so little. Increasing evidence suggests that vaginal birth is advantageous and preferable for the majority of women. For the baby, too, normal labour is a positive experience, the benefits of which we are only beginning to discover.

Labour is almost always in two stages that can be termed the latent phase of labour and the active phase of labour.

The latent stage could last a few hours or up to a few days. It involves contractions, which, though just as important, are not those that will result in the birth of your baby. These early and sometimes quite painful contractions are designed to prepare your baby, your uterus and your birth canal for the active phase of labour. During the latent phase, necessary physical changes take place: the birth canal softens and the cervix starts to ripen and become thinner, preparing to stretch and open with the onset of increasingly stronger and more frequent contractions. This degree of preparation has to be achieved in order that the next phase can begin. It frequently happens that a woman, being unaware that there are two phases of labour, naturally assumes that these contractions are the onset of active labour. Where a woman has access to a dedicated caregiver, she can seek reassurance that these contractions are a normal part of her body's preparation. This, in turn, will re-establish the confidence she has in her body and enable her to trust her inner feelings.

Active labour is when contractions become regular, increasingly frequent, stronger and more lengthy, lasting possibly as long as 60 seconds or more, and with the baby progressing through the birth canal while the cervix dilates at its own pace. Cervical dilatation is very often achieved quite rapidly towards the end of the first stage of active labour and is not necessarily the gradual process that is expected although both are normal. In normal labour, dilatation will facilitate the further descent of the baby and even at this stage of advanced labour, time constraints should not apply unless a deviation from norm has occurred.

This active stage of labour is also referred to as the first stage of labour. Many textbooks suggest that at the end of the first stage of labour and once a woman has achieved full dilatation of her cervix (the neck of the womb dilating to 10 cm in diameter), then the second stage (the pushing stage) is ready to begin. An experienced midwife attending a woman in advancing first stage of labour will, by experience, possess the ability to observe and to determine if the mother has transitioned into second-stage labour, at which point she may experience an increasingly overwhelming desire to push.

Prior to this pushing stage of labour it is not uncommon for a woman to enjoy a "rest and be thankful" stage, when the contractions fade and occasionally stop altogether. This breather allows a woman time to rest, to eat, or even to sleep, providing that she and her unborn baby are well. Should this happen, it is often a short respite of several minutes, but occasionally it can be as long as a few hours.

The final stage of labour is when the uterus reduces dramatically in size following the birth of the baby. This reduction leads to the shearing off of the placenta from the uterine wall, creating an amazing phenomenon known as the living ligature. While a certain amount of blood loss is totally normal and expected, this is nature's way of minimizing maternal blood loss following the birth of a baby. The complete normality of this process continues as we simply wait for uterine contractions to return, confirming the fact that the placenta and membranes have separated and are ready to be born by the maternal effort of gentle pushing. Once again, time should not be a factor during this important third stage, unless a problem arises.

The medicalization of normal pregnancy, coupled with the time and resource constraints imposed upon women within "the system", has led to a foreshortening of what nature intended. This often results in unnecessary complications and a less than satisfactory birth experience, often denying women any opportunity to touch base with their instincts.

THE SIGNS THAT LABOUR HAS BEGUN

As you near the end of your pregnancy, you will begin to anticipate any signs, however slight, that your baby may be ready to arrive. You also may appreciate subtle changes in your body. The onset of labour can manifest itself in many ways, and will be different for each woman. As you progress along the path of normal pre-labour, your body may be showing signs that it is making progress towards the long anticipated birth of your baby. These indications may be slow, subtle and unobtrusive, or they may be more obvious. You may even experience a degree of discomfort as the physical and psychological aspects of late pregnancy affect your body's normal balance.

If it hasn't before, your baby's head should descend lower into your pelvis, giving you more space to breathe. Any heartburn symptoms you may have will be eased, and you'll no longer feel uncomfortably full after a meal. However, once your baby's head is settled in your pelvis, you'll probably need to pass water and have bowel movements more frequently because of the pressure that your baby is placing on your bladder and bowels. If you are in early labour, prostaglandins, which are the body chemicals released at this time, may even trigger episodes of loose bowel movements. The relaxation of your joints and ligaments may make your pubic bones and back ache, and you may

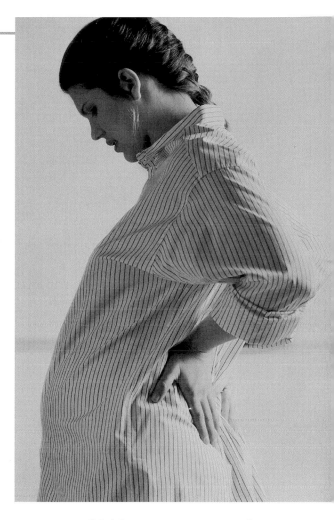

Many women will feel their contractions most strongly in their backs; this is most likely to occur if the back of their baby's head is pressing against their spine. Your birth attendant may be able to advise pain-relieving positions.

experience sharp twinges as your baby presses down on your pelvic floor. Your legs and feet may swell due to the compression of pelvic blood vessels. As your cervix softens, you may experience increased vaginal secretions. This discharge is usually like egg white, but it can be tinged pink. A yellow or frothy discharge may signal an infection, so you should report it to your healthcare provider.

NESTING INSTINCT

If you haven't experienced it before, you can find yourself seized with a sudden desire to empty drawers, clear out closets and scrub the house from top to bottom. This is what's known as the "nesting instinct", an inbuilt maternal urge to prepare the home for the imminent arrival of your baby. While you may want to make the most of this burst of energy, take care not to overdo it. You need to conserve your strength for labour.

THE SHOW

You may become aware of a plug of mucus, often bloodstained. This "show" can occur days before the onset of established labour, but it is a sure sign that your cervix is ripening and preparing to thin and stretch, rupturing the long-established network of fine blood vessels that exist at the neck of the uterus.

PAINLESS CONTRACTIONS

Braxton Hicks contractions are a naturally occurring phenomenon, often beginning as early as 20 weeks. They may become stronger as labour becomes imminent, further making you aware of your body's physical preparation.

BREAKING OF THE WATERS

Another indication of imminent labour is the rupture of the membranes or the bag of waters that has surrounded your baby during your pregnancy, endeavouring to keep him safe from trauma, infection and probably much more that we have yet to discover. As yet we are unsure as to the reason why the membranes occasionally rupture before the onset of labour. This can present you with a potential dilemma. The fact is that your unborn baby now has potentially lost his protection against infection. Should you remain at home, monitoring your temperature with surveillance by your midwife with the use of appropriate modern technology as and when indicated to confirm maternal and

HOW THE HEAD ENGAGES

Usually, in the weeks before birth, but occasionally hours or even minutes before delivery, your baby's head will descend or drop into your pelvis. Your midwife can measure the depth.

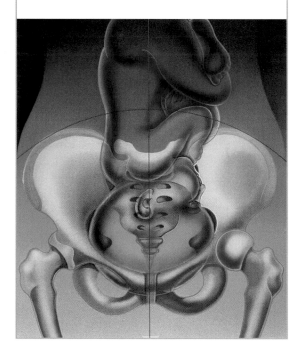

I remember caring for a first-time mother whose fore-waters broke when she was 37 weeks pregnant. She monitored her temperature and pulse three times daily and was encouraged to report any deviation from normal. I visited daily to monitor her baby's wellbeing, monitoring his heartbeat and using my hand-held sonic aid. With the mother's permission I obtained a vaginal swab to confirm the presence or absence of any infection at that time. Three days later, without any apparent complication following the rupture of her membranes, the mother and I discussed the options available. She considered them all in detail and decided to make use of hospital technology in order to confirm, as she felt, all was well with her baby. The scan and CTG monitor showed all to be quite normal. Although the doctor on duty was bound by hospital protocol to explain the "risks" of returning home and resisting induction of labour, she felt that her decision to return home was a safe option but fully understood the doctor's perspective. Another two days elapsed before she finally progressed into normal established labour and birthed a beautiful baby daughter. We agreed to take a precautionary measure of swabbing the baby's ears, nose and throat, and all proved to be negative for signs of infection. That little girl now has two little sisters, all born safely at home.

fetal wellbeing until the spontaneous onset of labour? Or should you follow protocol, whereby you will be granted a limited amount of time (which will vary from hospital to hospital) before induction is initiated? My belief is that the former is more preferable, for once you are admitted to the hospital the risk of infection soars, in fact much more so than at home. Naturally, if there is a complication affecting either your safety or that of your baby, your feelings will be even more significant. In these circumstances your instincts will be heightened, and they should reinforce your natural ability to monitor your unborn baby's wellbeing. Heeding them, you will subsequently be able to decide how best to harmonize your instincts with any modern technology available.

KNOWING YOU ARE IN LABOUR

Appreciating when labour has started is sometimes very difficult for a first-time mother. If you're one, you've never encountered these feelings before so you don't have the benefit of experience. In fact, all you have to rely on is the knowledge you have acquired from your sources, the carers responsible for you, and your instinct. The emotions surrounding the end of pregnancy can cause significant turbulence for all those involved, as each and every one has her (and his) own expectations. This is the point at which you particularly need the reassurance of a qualified professional who will offer an honest and unbiased appraisal of what you may be experiencing. If you are confident that all is well and appreciate that your baby is soon to be born, you will remain calm. Your labour has begun in whichever way nature has deemed appropriate.

Many mothers consider that they have laboured for days, unaware that, on occasion, nature requires considerable time to prepare your body for the crucial phase that will end with the birth of your baby. Remembering that the all-important latent stage of labour is not uncommon, and has to be achieved before the next phase can begin, should keep you sane! If you are aware that your body is designed to cope with this type of labour, and you believe it to be true, you can be totally and instinctively in control. As a consequence, this will reduce the likelihood that you may become nervous, frightened, and even doubt that you have the ability to cope.

The ability to predict when labour will begin is impossible! Nature is clever and keeps you guessing. It is possible to start contracting at regular intervals and then for your body to take a natural break. First-time mothers may be tempted to reach for their stopwatches, and begin to chart the timing of each contraction. My advice is not to focus too much on the frequency of contractions until they reach a point where they require total concentration – that is, they prevent you from doing anything else. Should you still be able to continue normal activities while experiencing contractions, then it is almost certain that you are not in active labour. There is time enough for your partner to get paper, pen, and stop-watch when total concentration is required to cope with each contraction. This is labour and will, sooner or later, result in your baby's birth.

Of all the women whose childbirths I have attended, I can honestly say that each one was unique with no two the same.

INTERVENTIONAL PRACTICES

Sweeping the membranes (see box, opposite), along with routine vaginal examinations, are, in my opinion, both unnecessary and invasive in most instances as well as being quite painful procedures. Women often recall them as the worst parts of their labours. Not only is this intervention physically discomforting, but more importantly it can have a very negative psychological impact on a woman. How often have I heard women recount stories in which following a routine vaginal examination during their latent phase of labour, they were told: "You are only one/two/three centimetres dilated". Even more demoralizing is to be told: "No you are not in labour. We suggest that you go home and return when contractions are stronger and closer together." A pregnant woman's mind is such a powerful asset that it should be encouraged at all times.

Any interference with this process will inhibit the timing and, therefore, the progress of labour. Talk to any experienced midwife, and she will assure you that discreet, non-invasive observation of a mother in labour will almost always provide significant evidence to gauge her progress. If, on the other hand, you request a vaginal examination, or accept that there is an obstetric indication requiring such a procedure that you have understood and agreed to, this can indicate that you are prepared mentally and emotionally for such a procedure. In this case, you will be as relaxed as possible and, more importantly, you will be in control of what is happening.

This book has a very simple message: we all have instincts and they can give us direction, if we listen to them. Childbirth is the ideal opportunity to use your instincts. Just as the mind and body are finely tuned during pregnancy, so are they working deeply together during the birth itself.

SWEEPING THE MEMBRANES

This is a procedure often performed by a midwife or obstetrician. It involves placing an examining finger inside the neck of the womb in an endeavour to peel the accessible membrane away from the wall of the uterus while also stretching the cervix in an attempt to hasten the onset of active labour. I don't believe it "works". Even when I did believe it to be of benefit to a woman, I found it simply intensified the already painful contractions to such a degree that the mother required early pain relief even before labour was established and her energy levels were becoming depleted. So, I no longer recommend this procedure. Only now are we becoming increasingly aware of the tremendous sensitivity of the cervix and the impact that any interference may have. By respecting the powerful influence that it can have on a woman's progress in labour, myself and other professionals are more concerned to monitor a woman through observation, rather than visible intervention.

TIMING OF LABOUR

Labour is so variable as to duration and how it manifests that it is hard to generalize; it shouldn't, therefore, be the basis upon which to measure personal experience. The advice that I offer mothers in my care is to prepare themselves for active labour to last approximately 24 hours, being one special day out of the whole of their lives. There will always be exceptions to "normal" labour – a woman who spends two to three hours and one who spends three days are not experiences we witness every day. The most exceptional labour that I have personally witnessed was one where a woman experienced five days of intermittent labour. She felt safe and secure at home and as mother and baby were well, there was no need to contemplate transferring to the hospital immediately. However, she did eventually decide she was ready to go into the hospital and here she had a normal delivery. This illustrates that a woman can remain in control even when stretched to the ultimate lengths with which her body can cope.

The variability of labour makes it difficult to advise a woman how best to manage it, especially her first experience. Predicting anything is virtually impossible, so the best that her caregiver can do is to prepare a woman by showing her where and what information is available, and by providing her with a calm and consistent sounding board upon which she is free to voice her questions, doubts, hopes and fears. The goal should be to increase her own knowledge and wisdom about the beautiful mechanism of labour and birth, encouraging her to listen to, and trust in, her body and her instincts.

A woman's psychological and emotional approach to labour will not only influence the progress of labour but also, in most cases, influence the outcome of how she births her baby. A woman who has made personal choices during her pregnancy and has been pivotal in the preparation of her labour and birth, is likely to achieve the most fulfilment – provided her wishes are respected. This is true both of a woman wishing a completely drug-free, natural labour and birth, as well as a woman who believes she will require all the pain relief available. The former feels safe in the knowledge that her body was designed for pregnancy, labour and birth, and thus the pain of contractions will be met by her body's natural ability to cope with and manage pain. The latter feels safe in the knowledge that there are drugs available to help her body overcome a situation for which she may feel fear. Both women are following the driving forces of their instincts and, if allowed to progress as desired, both will feel fulfilled in that they have maintained control of their experiences and made choices that allowed them to feel safe and assured.

STRATEGIES FOR PAIN

The pain experienced in labour is also unique to each woman. It will vary from woman to woman, and in the same woman may vary from birth to birth, and in a single labour may move from one position to another as labour progresses.

The key to dealing with discomfort is to be mentally prepared and to try to establish ways of calming and focussing your mind. Everyone has a different pain threshold and varying ways of dealing with pain, so what works for your friend may not work for you. However, every woman has been born with the ability to birth their babies, so you can enter the birthing experience with confidence and anticipation, rather than fear and trepidation.

MAINTENANCE OF NORMAL ACTIVITIES

My advice to mothers, especially those approaching labour for the first time, is to continue normal activity in early labour. If early labour occurs at night, attempting to sleep or rest will provide you with a source of strength that will prove useful during the later active stage. If labour begins during the day, attempting to maintain your normal pattern or routine will help to focus your mind on activities other than the contractions. Your body will dictate how much or how little you should be eating or drinking, so don't artificially restrict your intake. However, with the progress of labour your body's ability to digest food diminishes and you will naturally not feel hungry. Labour contractions often accelerate as night falls, which may well be due to differing levels of hormones at night than day. Giving birth requires high levels of calories. It is therefore important that you have energy-giving sustenance. Honey, bananas or high-energy drinks, will ensure that your body does not become depleted of much needed energy.

RHYTHMICAL BREATHING

Human nature dictates that we instinctively react to pain in a predictable way. When the human body is subjected to pain, for whatever reason and from whatever source, the reaction is usually to hold your breath until the pain begins to subside. Ordinarily, this reaction is not of any great significance or consequence, but not so in labour. As a result of breath-holding, your muscles will be deprived of vital oxygen and the pain will increase. The uterus itself is a large, powerful muscle – and one of the most amazing muscles in the female body. A woman in advancing labour needs to be gently or quietly reminded with each strong contraction to relax and breathe in order to make a measurable and positive impact on her labour. Rhythmical breathing throughout the increasingly strong contractions will enhance her body's ability to relax and progress. Using steady breathing to focus your mind on the ebb and flow of the contractions will help your body to manage the pain.

The pain-relieving abilities of endorphins are enhanced in a relaxed and fearless mother who trusts her body to perform as nature intended.

HYDROTHERAPY

Water often brings another dimension to labour. Not only can it be used as an effective relaxant during the early stages, it can also be used as a location for the birth itself. Many women have an instinctive affinity for water immersion. Research has proven beyond doubt that a mother who chooses to access water for her labour and/or birth will benefit

Cindy was two weeks beyond her "due date" when her labour began spontaneously. By the time I arrived at the house, Cindy was having strong contractions every five minutes and they were lasting over a minute. She was pacing to and fro, dropping to her knees with each contraction and breathing through them, needing only words of encouragement from her husband, Peter, and me. Cindy was desperate to enter the warm inviting pool and asked me if she could. I readily agreed as I was there to support her own instinctive behaviour. Her labour was hard and relentless but my frequent observations showed Cindy and her baby were both well. After six hours in the pool and the labour continuing normally albeit slowly, I suggested to Cindy that vacating the pool and allowing gravity to play a part might encourage more progress. Cindy agreed. She knelt over a stack of pillows, coping magnificently with her demanding labour. She had lots of encouragement and reassurance, as well as hot towels applied to her lower back where the pain was greatest.

Vacating the pool and allowing gravity to take effect did the trick. Cindy progressed beautifully into the second stage of labour after six hours on "dry land". She once again climbed into the pool, allowing the warm water to envelope her seemingly exhausted body. After another three hours of instinctively harmonizing her strength with the overwhelmingly expulsive contractions, Cindy birthed her 9 lb 3 oz son. With the cord still pulsating, and at Cindy's invitation, Peter joined his wife and newborn son in the pool.

from a measurable pain-relieving effect. Allowing the warm water to surround you will help your body to relax and yield to your own powerful pain relievers, the endorphins.

I feel that constraints as to when and for how long a mother uses water in her labour and birth are inappropriate. Instinctively a mother will know when she wishes to immerse herself in water and for how long she remains. I have never known a mother who has refused to leave the pool in the event of a complication. Once in the birthing pool, a labouring mother becomes more self-sufficient, as the balmy warmth of the water often replaces the need for intermittent back massage, or any other physical support she may have needed.

Our body's natural ability to deal with pain is quite amazing. In response to increasingly strong contractions, endorphin production is triggered, and, as labour advances, increases to keep pace.

TENS

Endorphins work in the opposite way to adrenaline, which is stimulated by the body when you start to panic or are put under unwelcome pressure. If you have ever wondered what a TENS (Trans Electrical Nerve Stimulation) machine does, it stimulates certain points on the body to help increase the endorphins. It is a set of two pads, which are attached to a woman's lower back and through which an electrical pulse is delivered with increasing intensity during labour, as controlled by the mother. This is why it is recommended that a TENS machine is used as early in labour as possible, in order that you give the endorphins time to build up sufficiently. Many women find this a very useful form of non-drug pain relief: having to acknowledge a contraction and focussing the mind on activating the TENS machine can be quite effective in diverting the pain. My slight concern with this potential method of pain relief is the possible premature messages created by the mind that labour has begun. In other words, should you have a prolonged labour in which you monitor each contraction from the early stages, psychologically and emotionally it may feel to you that your labour is longer than it really is. Remembering that labour has two phases (see page 115) and endeavouring to apply the TENS at the appropriate time in active labour will ensure maximum effectiveness of its pain-reducing ability.

GAS AND AIR

Entonox – 50 percent Oxygen and 50 percent Nitrous Oxide gas – can also be useful in active labour. Using either a mask or a mouthpiece attached by tubing to the Entonox, you will inhale deeply through your mouth. The deep breathing should commence as your contractions begin. You continue to breathe in this way for a number of breaths or until the contraction has peaked. The concentration of anaesthetic will make you feel floaty but as the gas and air are self-administered, it will be impossible for you to become anaesthetized. Your hand, which is holding the mask or mouthpiece, will simply relax or fall away. Having experienced this method of pain relief, some mothers like the effects. Conversely some do not, as they feel a loss of control. The effects of gas and air are short-lived, harmless and non-accumulative, thus providing effective pain relief for a mother advancing in normal labour.

It is important to understand that as soon as intervention is suggested, you will be losing control of your own ability to birth your baby and passing the control, and in some instances the outcome, over to someone else.

PETHIDINE

This is an opioid painkiller and is administered by an intramuscular injection into a labouring mother. Opioids bind to the same receptors in the brain as endorphins, and thus restrict the transmission of pain signals from cell to cell. For many, pethidine is a controversial drug, and is probably used less today than it was a generation ago when epidurals were in their infancy and it was the drug of choice. As a method of pain relief, pethidine is physically less invasive and its effects more immediate than an epidural.

Once administered, the influence of pethidine cannot be reversed, and the effects usually subside within two to four hours. A mother who has received a dose becomes quiet, subdued, and often disassociated from her labour, unable to interact with her carers and therefore unable to participate effectively in decision making. It has been established that pethidine, administered to a mother in labour, can be detected in traceable quantities in her baby for at least two weeks after the injection. It is also known that pethidine adversely affects a baby by depressing his respiratory effort at birth, which, in turn, often impacts on his feeding ability. Some midwives, observing a woman perceived to be struggling with her advancing labour, will recommend the administration of pethidine in an attempt to ease the pain. I, however, seldom use pethidine.

EPIDURAL ANALGESIA

This is another method of pain relief in labour, which can only be administered by a qualified anaesthetist. It is a sterile procedure. Initially, the mother-to-be is usually required to sit with her back rounded in order to separate the vertebrae, so that the anaesthetist can identify the injection site before the procedure begins. First local anaesthetic is injected into the proposed site and then a needle is inserted in an attempt to locate the epidural space in front of the spinal cord. Once the epidural space is located, the anaesthetist will introduce a fine catheter through which the pain-relieving drug will be administered. He or she will then remove the needle, leaving the catheter firmly taped in place. A test dose of the drug will then be administered via the catheter and, if there are no adverse effects, the full top-up dose will be given.

Prior to commencing the procedure the anaesthetist will always make you aware of the risks involved. These may include partial or total failure to relieve the pain due to a variety of reasons. There is also a minor risk of inadvertently puncturing the spinal cord by advancing beyond the epidural space. This would allow the cerebrospinal fluid within to leak out and may cause a blinding headache. You would have to lie flat for about 48 hours before gradual mobilization would be allowed. In extreme circumstances, maladministration of an epidural can result in paralysis to the mother.

A successful epidural will eliminate the pain of contractions. This is a great source of comfort to many women, and has helped to quash the fear of giving birth for a lot of women. Timed appropriately, an epidural can facilitate the progress of what might become a complicated labour. However, it is important that you become aware, before labour begins, of the potential impact this method may have on the actual birthing outcome. Firstly, this procedure requires having an intravenous infusion (a drip) in place before and during the administration of the epidural to counterbalance any falls in maternal blood pressure that may result from the epidural.

Because an epidural numbs the nerves and therefore the pain, it is actually quite difficult to feel the surge of the contractions. Many women can only see when their uterus is contracting by looking at a monitor. This is usually applied for the duration of labour and means that physical movement is dramatically reduced. This restriction of movement, in turn, can have a dramatic effect on your progress. In the second stage of labour, you need to be able to really feel the strength of the expulsive sensation and use your total body force to birth your baby. Not only does the horizontal position preferred for the procedure impede gravity's natural force, but the lack of sensation caused by the epidural may reduce the intensity of the pushing sensation, resulting in an instrumental delivery, such as ventouse, forceps, or even caesarean section. This is because your body would not have been able to push your baby out as efficiently as it would have had if you had been in an

Babies birth themselves; mothers deliver their babies; midwives simply have hands outstretched, ready to catch the baby safely.

Caroline, a first-time mother, had adapted her spare room in preparation for her forthcoming labour. She had furnished it with a pool, a bean bag, a large inflatable ball, a swing and a bed. She began to spontaneously labour well beyond her due date. It was a wholesome, progressive labour though slow and steady. But 21 hours later, Caroline was saying "I can't do this, I need help!" Caroline was confident that I would take heed of her instinctive decision, even though she was approaching second stage labour. I arranged hospital transfer as Caroline had decided. Knowing that she was in control and that help was at hand, she relaxed and was soon in the glorious pushing stage of her active labour, progressing beautifully and eventually birthed a lovely baby daughter.

If a mother in labour reaches the stage when she believes that she is struggling, the support and information that she receives will directly influence the outcome; more often than not it's the resolve that results in her saying "I can do it" – and more often than not – she does!

upright position with full awareness and participation in your second stage contractions. The post-delivery side effects of an epidural include difficulty in passing urine after the catheter is removed, and a delay of several hours following discontinuation of the epidural before sensation in your legs is regained.

Awareness is increasing as to the questionable over-use of this invasive method of pain relief for normal labour. An increasing number of hospitals are no longer providing epidurals on demand. In fact, some units have no epidural service at all. As a result, those mothers looking to birth their babies in those units obviously do not expect to have an epidural.

CHOOSING WHAT'S BEST FOR YOU

Balancing the advantages and the disadvantages of the different forms of pain relief is an important part of your preparations for birth. Your decision needs to be understood and respected by your birth partner and carers. Whatever method of pain relief you choose, this should be through informed choice and in response to the messages your instinct is sending. Of course, there may be unforeseen circumstances as well as the inevitable experience of the unknown (especially when it comes to individual pain threshold) and these may well require immediate further decisions to be made. Yet even these decisions should be based on information and knowledge, as they will be very important for your birth psychology and personal self-fulfilment. Any woman who feels that she can no longer continue in her labour without effective pain relief must have her decision respected. However, such a woman may well be looking to her trusted midwife for guidance in her decision-making. The desire for help often arises when a woman is reaching the end of first stage labour, when her cervix is almost fully dilated, and her contractions are at their most powerful but as yet are not expulsive. This stage is often referred to as "transition", and an experienced birth practitioner will be able to draw upon her expertise to reassure the mother that she is actually experiencing a very positive part of labour and that her baby is imminent. This information is

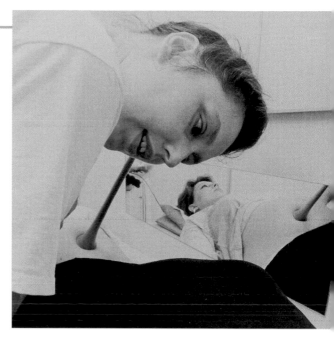

Your birth practitioner can quickly assess your baby's wellbeing by listening to his heartbeat with a Pinard's stethoscope rather than using invasive vaginal investigations.

often just what's needed to impart inspiration and optimism, and many women are then able to call on another source of strength that carries them through.

LABOURING WITH LOVE

An experienced midwife can assess to a high degree of accuracy how the mother in her care is progressing during labour by quiet observation, nonverbal communication, and often without the need for vaginal examinations. She can do this without any intrusion into the mother's space save only to monitor the baby's heart-rate, using a hand-held instrument called a sonic aid. Some mothers refuse even this intrusion into the baby's sanctuary, and prefer their midwives to use the Pinard's stethoscope (a trumpet-like instrument). Observation of the mother's pulse rate will tell the midwife how the mother's body is responding to the demands of labour.

Assessing the progress of labour is only part of a skilled midwife's role. She can draw from her accumulated knowledge to suggest achievable goals based on her assessment of the progress of your labour, and without you becoming distressed and feeling that you are losing control.

Imagine you, an informed mother-to-be, as an active participant in the decision-making process and in control of the direction in which your labour is heading. You will

A healthy labouring woman has the strength of a lion.

decide when and when not to take nourishment, either food or drink, for your body is designed to react instinctively if sustenance is required. You labour quietly with loved ones of your choosing. You feel emotionally strong. Your body is able to react totally naturally, producing endorphins in increasing amounts in accordance with the status of your labour. You can relax between contractions, and often feel very comfortable as you adopt a safe position that allows you to recoup and re-engage your mind with your body.

Once you're in labour you will instinctively stand, kneel or squat in response to your contractions. You may also walk around during the early stages. You will not choose to lie flat on your back. More active birthing positions abate the intensity of contractions and they also are more beneficial to your baby, resulting in maximum oxygen levels to the baby as blood flow to the uterus is unrestricted. You may also use a support to help you adopt a natural labouring position, such as the side of the bed, a birthing ball, or your chosen birthing partner. If your energy becomes depleted, however, you may benefit from lying down on your left side. This position will not impede the progress of labour.

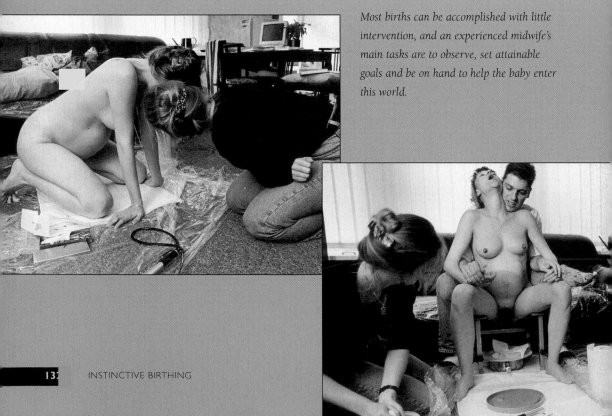

Most births can be accomplished with little intervention, and an experienced midwife's main tasks are to observe, set attainable goals and be on hand to help the baby enter this world.

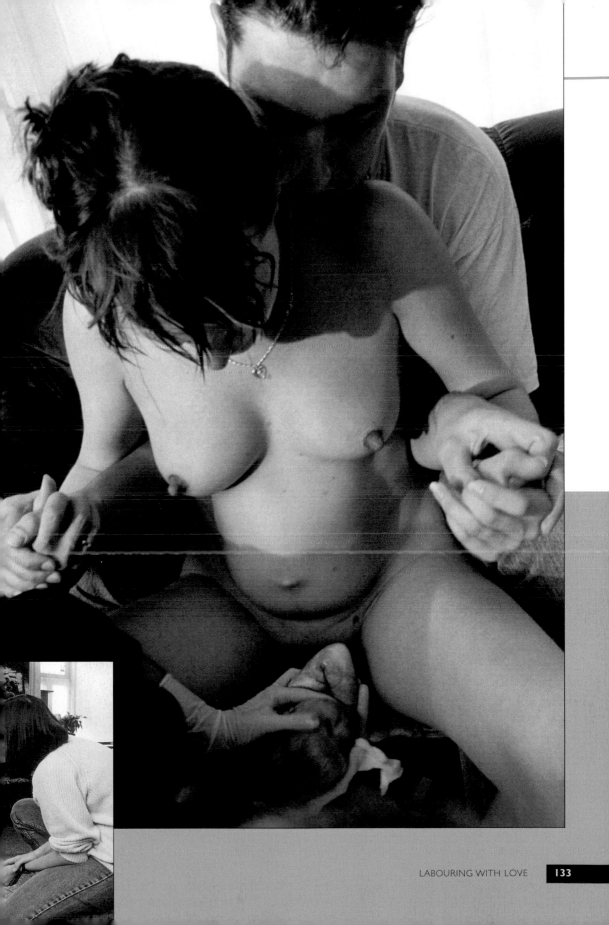

✳ The most incredible case of a mother confidently trusting her body was Elena. She began her labour on a Sunday evening. The next 24 hours saw her progress to 4 cm cervical dilatation. She went in and out of her birthing pool and was sleeping during the many "rest and be thankful phases". I became involved by way of relieving her attending midwife, who'd been with her from the beginning of labour, so she could get some sleep. Elena continued to labour on and off until the following Friday; during all of this time she felt safe, confident and determined that she could safely birth her baby. Both myself and the attending midwife, as well as an obstetrician who volunteered to be a birth supporter, were able to reassure her that although incredibly slow by any standards, Elena was safely progressing in her labour. After being in and out of labour for over five days, Elena finally decided that a hospital transfer was desirable, exclaiming "Enough is enough!" Within a few short hours following her admission, and without any intervention, Elena delivered her healthy baby daughter. We will never know why Elena's journey to motherhood took so long, but I am so very happy to say that mother and baby are well.

ADVANCED LABOUR

Once you are in advanced labour, the variety of positions that you may adopt are great, and will always be prompted by your progress and environment. When you feel completely safe and secure in your birthing environment, you will adopt positions that are the most favourable – those that not only allow you to move freely and without inhibition, but also will encourage the flow of hormones that facilitate the labour process. You may find soothing music and scented candles help in making your surroundings comforting.

As the birth approaches even nearer, you may need more frequent, quietly spoken reassurances from the person in whom you have entrusted your care. You will be free to listen intently and to respond to all your innermost feelings. Whether in water or not, it is at this moment that you will totally yield to your body's silent voice. Advancing into the second stage of labour, no woman birthing her baby and using her heightened instincts should be given instructions on how to perform this truly miraculous activity.

Your baby has to negotiate an incredible path in order to be born. This journey requires time and patience, so progress might be slow. Nature and your emotional, psychological and spiritual states will influence this progress. It is inevitable that a degree of impatience will surround the labour and birth but, providing you and your baby are healthy, and your baby is making progress on his journey, then time constraints should not apply. Throughout labour, and even occasionally at any stage in established labour, your contractions may diminish. View this as valuable time in which to eat or sleep or both. There is no need for haste. Problems often occur when a mother's labour or birth is accelerated without good reason.

THE FINAL STAGES

At any moment during your labour, your membranes might rupture if they have not already done so. As the transition approaches, you will feel a different sensation and, in recognition of these powerful and increasingly expulsive contractions, you may announce to your carers that your baby is coming. You will continue to work instinctively and quietly with your body. Maybe the quiet earthy moans you have uttered during contractions now increasingly become deeper sounds or even roars. How clever is nature, for this instinctive roar, combined with your overwhelming desire to push, will reduce the possibility of trauma to your birth canal and perineum. This is another reason why the birth of a baby is not an event to be orchestrated, for this stage of your labour, as with every other stage, has been finely tuned by nature to ensure a healthy mother.

As your baby's head crowns, you will experience what midwives aptly describe as the "ring of fire". This is the vagina and perineum stretching and yielding to accommodate the emerging head.

Too many mothers are advised that their cervixes are fully dilated and instructed to begin pushing. As a result, they will use vital energy attempting to expedite the births of their babies when their contractions as yet are not expulsive and their bodies are simply not ready. Even at this late stage in labour, contractions can, and sometimes do, fade away in their strength and frequency and, occasionally, may stop

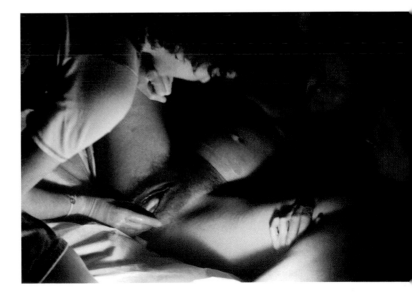

altogether. Providing you and your baby are healthy, any rests of nature should be regarded as normal. Respecting a labouring mother's body should be mandatory. Occasionally, although in the second stage of labour, a mother will not experience expulsive contractions until her baby's head is visible.

Once your baby's head crowns, you will then, in the position of your choice, deliver your baby. Similarly, nature's lifeline, the umbilical cord, should be left untouched until it has ceased pulsation; only then should it be clamped and cut, an activity that can be performed by you or your partner. Your baby receives all the oxygen and nourishment he requires right up until the time the cord has ceased pulsating and is cut.

THIRD-STAGE LABOUR

As and when nature indicates, the third stage of labour will begin and you will experience occasional contractions. Slowly the placenta and the membranes will be delivered and, if you wish, there is no reason why you should not assist their birth by holding the end of the umbilical cord and applying gentle traction.

The entire process of labour and birth is amazing in the extreme. Nature has designed the female human body to bring forth babies, a process about which we know and understand relatively so very little. However, what we do know, and what can be attested by anyone fortunate enough to witness the miracle of birth, is the sheer and profound fulfilment etched on a mother's face when she delivers her child. As Thomas Verny says: "Providing the newborn with a warm, reassuring environment does make a difference because the child is very aware of how he is born. He senses gentleness, softness and a caring touch, and he responds to them much as he senses and responds in quite a different way to the bright lights, electrical beeps and cold, impersonal atmosphere that are so often associated with a medical birth."

VULNERABILITY OF WOMEN IN LABOUR

I believe very strongly that newly pregnant, first-time mothers, for whom "the system" represents the core of their care and which may be the only choice they believe they have, are placed in a very vulnerable position. Decades of disempowerment created by increased medical intervention in normal pregnancies and media influence, have led to few newly pregnant women believing they have the fundamental right to challenge what "the system" provides in terms of antenatal care. Even if a mother feels that she may want to explore alternative routes, she is seldom encouraged to do so, not only by those advising her but also by her partner, who may feel safer within the boundaries and norms established by the status quo.

While I, too, have practiced within "the system" and know there are many exceptional individuals who cherish the ethics and values we all aspire to, the sad reality

✱ Eagerly awaiting the birth of their first baby and having enjoyed an uncomplicated pregnancy, Emily and her partner were advised at 41 weeks that their baby was "small-for-dates". This was confirmed by ultrasound scan and induction of labour was strongly recommended, as it was feared the baby was not thriving. The couple was devastated by the news; their plan for their baby's birth was for it to be as free of intervention and drugs as possible. They now faced a dilemma in that their unborn baby's wellbeing was in question. After a couple of days' searching for the right answer, they reluctantly agreed to the induction and it took place. Emily's cervix was deemed to be unfavourable and, over the course of two days at regular intervals, the prostin gel was inserted into her vagina around her cervix in an attempt to increase its favourability. During this time Emily and her partner paced up and down the hospital corridors in a vain attempt to stimulate the natural onset of labour, but to no avail. By day three and with the cervix artificially favourable, the next step in induction was embarked upon. During a vaginal examination, the membranes were artificially ruptured followed by the siting of an intravenous drip with the oxytocic drug added. Emily was still valiantly attempting to facilitate her body to react instinctively in spite of this unwelcome onslaught. She was able to resist the offers of pain relief, including an epidural. By day four, however, she finally resigned herself to what she perceived to be the inevitable – an epidural and, as she expected, a caesarean section soon followed. She was finally delivered of a healthy baby boy weighing 7 lbs 5 oz. It took Emily many weeks of spirited determination to establish breastfeeding, which she happily continued to do for a whole year. After three years of healing the emotional wounds of this birth, she is pregnant once more and planning a home birth with an independent midwife.

in many cases is that lip service is paid to the words "informed choice". The few women who choose to explore alternative options tend to be more in tune with their bodies and often quite assertive, especially if they're first-time mothers. As a woman's pregnancy advances toward her labour, her vulnerability increases and this reaches its height once labour begins. To mitigate these circumstances, a woman would need to have been fortunate enough to have developed a trusting relationship with her caregiver and that her history, hopes, fears and ideals are fully understood and respected during labour and birth. There are the lucky few for whom this ideal is a reality and who are able to applaud "the system" for delivering a service that supported their aspirations of birth.

Unfortunately, the majority of women arrive at the delivery suite and are met by strange faces who, for the sake of efficiency and safety, will be keen to pigeonhole them into the standard patient model of care. And the likelihood is that this involves a simple request to the woman to lie on a bed while a monitor is attached to her abdomen to determine the baby's wellbeing and to establish the strength of contractions. Thus commences the loss of maternal control and the

Satisfying birthing memories are so powerful because they equip you for subsequent births, which you may look forward to with anticipation and excitement.

Cathy laboured spontaneously having reached term with her first pregnancy. Reading the labour and delivery notes as recorded by the attending midwife, one could imagine that it was the sort of labour that every mother would wish for, lasting no more than seven hours from beginning to end. For Cathy, however, the reality was quite different. She perceived it to be a nightmare experience as she felt completely out of control and subsequently developed postnatal depression. She waited three years before embarking on her next pregnancy. Her partner expressed the wish to be disassociated from any future event. For her second delivery, Cathy planned a home birth. At 42 weeks, having enjoyed a healthy pregnancy, she finally went into spontaneous labour. Her husband had no pressure whatsoever put upon him to play any part in the labour unless he so desired. He made tea and cared for their toddler daughter during what turned out to be a lengthy labour. The birthing atmosphere throughout was relaxed. Amazingly, Cathy's husband was dancing with his daughter on the birthing mat minutes before his 10 lb 3 oz son was born. Cathy did not develop postnatal depression this time around.

inevitable cascade of intervention. And all too often this is the experience of a woman in advancing labour who enters the delivery suite, having made her way from home where she has been coping well, using all her natural instincts and resources up until that moment in time. Any birth plan that may have been in place, carefully written by the woman realistically hoping to remain in control, often becomes redundant as she now succumbs to the pressure of convenience, protocols and policies.

INTERVENTION IN LABOUR

There are, of course, occasions when hospitals feel intervention is necessary and, unfortunately, it seems to be on the increase. Intervention can have quite a significant impact on your ability to birth your baby as you'd like.

The most obvious form of intervention is induction. Much importance is placed on the due date of the baby, so once this has passed most hospitals will begin to discuss induction dates. The policy on how far beyond their due dates women are allowed to go will vary from hospital to hospital and sometimes even from obstetrician to obstetrician.

As she agrees to the proposed artificially induced labour, a woman is seldom counselled about the process it involves. You may even reach the planned induction day only to be advised in your increased state of anxiety that no beds are available. This is a very distressing situation and probably far from the image you had of going into labour.

Induction of labour is an artificial method that encourages your uterus to start contracting. You will be told that it is essential to perform a vaginal examination in order to confirm the favourability (extent of dilation) of your cervix, and that this relevant information will influence the desired plan of action. This intrusion of a healthy, pregnant mother's body is just the beginning of a potential cascade of events guaranteed to erode little by little any control you may have had over your body. The induction process may even be presented to you in such a way that it could seem almost trivial and exceedingly tempting, for now you are heavy with child and anxious to see your newborn.

If your cervix is "unfavourable" (not dilated at all), it will be necessary for you to have a prostaglandin gel or pessary inserted vaginally. This will be repeated at regular intervals and sometimes over several days before the next stage can be embarked upon. Once your cervix becomes "favourable" (begins to dilate), a probe called an amnihook will be inserted into your vagina in an attempt to rupture the membranes surrounding your baby. Once the waters have ruptured, you will have a timescale within which your baby must be delivered. Part of the induction routine is the siting at this stage of an intravenous drip into which is added an artificial oxytocic drug designed to induce contractions. The increasingly painful contractions that follow are not a result of your body's own attempt to labour and birth, but merely the result of the vaginally administered prostaglandins or the oxytocic drip.

Induction of labour requires intermittent and sometimes continuous monitoring, restricting mobility. An artificially induced birth dramatically interferes with your own natural path into labour and birth: the induced contractions are not sufficient to influence the progress of labour on their own, neither is it possible for your vital endorphin response to be activated. As a result, you will experience a psychological and physical response to the sudden onset of painful contractions. Exposure to this type of labour often creates fear in a woman, which, in turn, may impact on the outcome. And you are likely to encounter more intervention, which will insidiously erode your ability to remain in control and behave instinctively. For example, when the pain from the induced contractions kicks in without the benefit of enhanced endorphins, many women will request artificial pain relief, such as an epidural.

Unless and until your own body responds and reacts favourably to the induction of labour, the timed progress will be unachievable and may result in instrumental birth. This type of birth would then be attributed to "failure to progress" rather than what should be termed "failed induction".

Induction also will be imposed if a woman's waters have broken naturally and labour has not commenced within a specified timescale, such as 24 or 48 hours. Hospital protocols or policies are likely to influence the management of this occurrence in order to prevent infection. Without doubt, the risk of infection is real; however, the reality of the hospital's parameters is questionable. For instance, your hospital may require you to attend as soon as possible in order that personnel may monitor your baby's heartbeat and inspect the colour of your vaginal fluid. This may be greenish, which could indicate that all might not be well with your baby. If all is well, however, then the hospital may allow you to return home – providing you attend for daily monitoring. After a certain length of time, as stated in the hospital's protocol, and with no signs of labour, the hospital will attempt to persuade you to submit to acceleration of labour.

I have known many women whose waters had broken and who had decided to wait for spontaneous labour to begin. They were vigilant about not exposing themselves to potential areas of infection, such as swimming pools, and went on safely to labour their babies as and when nature deemed it time.

Most women are unprepared for the relentless assault of medical intervention. Natural instincts will be suffocated by the activities of induction, one leading to another. The further tragedy is that many women, whose bodies refuse to respond to induction, are forced into having caesarean sections. It is only after the event that these mothers question the wisdom of those who, in the face of their ignorance of the process, guided them into submitting to an induction. "Never again" they vow. It is for this reason that I am hoping my book will form part of every first-time mother's library.

Of course it is easy for me, a midwife, to talk with confidence about the body's natural ability to go into labour, cope with pain, and help babies into this world. But for a first-time mother, lying on a bed within hospital, coping with an experience that is so emotionally and physically demanding, it is likely that your and your partner's confidence will slowly evaporate as your vulnerability increases and you unwittingly submit to the standard patient model of care.

Yet you have been preparing your body and mind for this moment; and if you are sufficiently strong to trust your instinct, your strongest resource, you will be amazed at what you can achieve. Your mind is your most powerful tool and a woman with a positive approach will feel energized and much more in control.

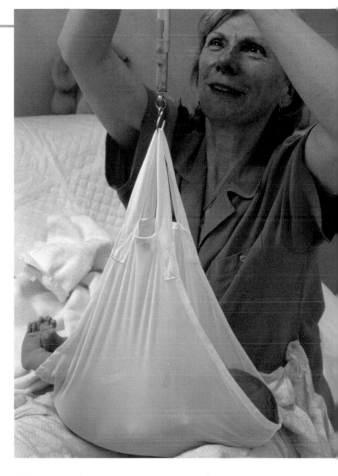

It's important for your emotional recovery that some time post delivery, you review your experience with your midwife. Often, a "textbook" labour for a carer is quite the opposite for the woman.

Often it is not until a woman has birthed her first baby that she reflects on how different the experience was from what she had expected and yet she feels fulfilled. She has done it and that gives her incredible strength, both emotional and psychological, even if she feels absolutely exhausted physically!

Every woman deserves to be able to cherish her birthing experience. I feel great satisfaction when I hear a mother recalling her first labour and birth as her most fulfilling experiences and being the best day of her life.

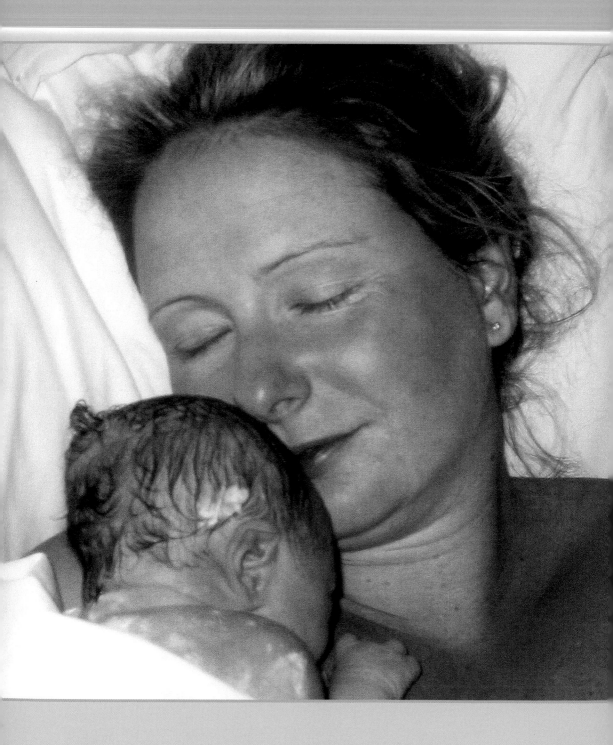

CHAPTER 8
Instinctive Continuum

✳ INSTINCTIVE CONTINUUM

During the few days and weeks following the birth of your baby you will experience many different and unfamiliar feelings. This is the case whether you are a first-time mother or have already been through labour and delivery previously. You will be recovering from the birth and reliving the event with yourself, your partner and many others. You will be learning how to look after your baby and trying to establish breastfeeding. You may be tired, even exhausted. Your baby now lies beside you close and safe. You have succeeded handsomely in one of life's miracles – the birth of a baby. The euphoria you are probably feeling now should remain for at least the first few days or more. These uplifting feelings are designed to ease the early demands of motherhood.

We perceive a newborn as acutely vulnerable and to some extent, he is. Yet nature has also equipped him with an incredibly strong instinct to survive as well as some survival behaviour. Combine that newborn's will to exist with his mother's overwhelming maternal instinct to protect and nurture him, and you should have the recipe for success. However, many factors influence that success and the degree to which it aspires.

CONTINUING YOUR PRE-BIRTH RELATIONSHIP

Before your baby's birth you will almost certainly have experienced gradual, intensifying feelings for the new and special life developing within you. Yet absolutely nothing can prepare you for that moment when you embrace your newborn for the first time. Much may depend on the ease or difficulty you may have experienced birthing your baby. Nevertheless, the gamut of emotions can be completely overwhelming.

Surprisingly, love may not be one of them. It is not exceptional for a mother to need quite a lengthy amount of time during which she gradually falls in love with her new baby. Mother love is not always like turning on a tap. Bear in mind that love is a powerful emotion and has different meanings to all people. Many mothers do not feel an instantaneous, overwhelming love for their newborn infants and consequently feel inadequate. As a result, they do not admit or confess their true feelings for fear of criticism. Concerned that something may go wrong, some women may subconsciously attempt to detach themselves from feeling strong surges of love until their babies are safe in their arms. Some may not have given too much thought to the initial emotional impact they may or may not experience when gazing at their newborns for the first time. Then there are those mothers who connect with their babies even before they are born, and the physical appearance of these little beings is further confirmation of the deep-rooted love that has grown between them.

Gazing at your newborn, you will bathe in the euphoria of your achievement.

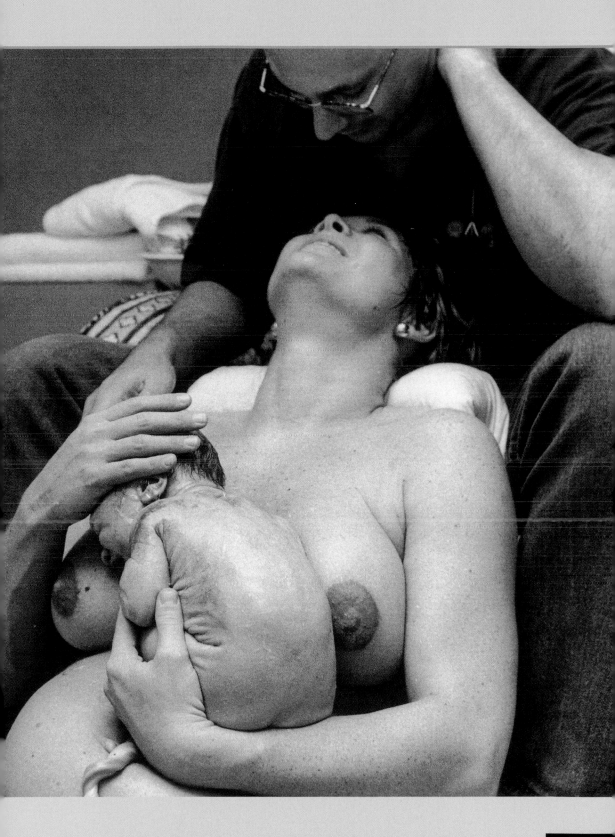

The ability to communicate and interact with your child in utero (see chapter five) may have consequences that we're only now beginning to understand.

Dr. Verny maintains that the prenatal relationship between mother and child is established not only at a physical level, but that there also are complex emotional and psychological responses occurring between the two. These will determine the path of much of their postnatal relationship building. By reading Verny you can glean further insight into the way in which your baby's continuum is established and nurtured both before and after birth. So much of it is based on deep and instinctive reactions.

Months before birth, mother and child were already beginning to mesh their rhythms and responses to each other. This pointed squarely to one conclusion: bonding after birth, which had always been studied as a singular and isolated phenomenon, was actually the continuation of a bonding process that began long before, in the womb.

Thomas Verny, *The Secret Life of the Unborn Child*

TAKING THE TIME TO GET ACQUAINTED

There is no hard and fast rule to bonding. It is, however, influenced dramatically by your own personal circumstances, which may or may not allow you to behave totally instinctively. Individuals who've had a poor relationship with their own parents will have to work harder at one than a couple who had warm, loving parents. Just as your pregnancy and birth were unique, so too will be the relationship you develop with your baby.

Before the onset of industrialization, when large extended families were the rule, and even as recent as one or two generations ago, new parents had the support of other family members who could relieve them of some of their day-to-day pressures, so that mothers, at least, could concentrate on caring for their new babies. Mother and baby spent precious time enjoying skin-to-skin contact and the baby was free to suckle at the breast as and when he needed sustenance or reassurance. Eager arms were always outstretched to cradle the little one, whose needs were so primitive. One's extended family supported and nurtured the new parents and baby, and, if necessary, any siblings.

Although few people today can depend on their extended families it is important that new mothers afford themselves time with their babies in order to get to know each other. Not so long ago, and still in some cultures today, a new mother was not expected to be up and about after a birth; she spent weeks lying in – attending just to her baby and being looked after by family or close friends.

Traditionally, during the first six weeks after birth, mothers and their babies "retired" from the world. Mothers could use the time to recuperate from the rigours of birth; babies would begin to learn to adapt to life outside the womb.

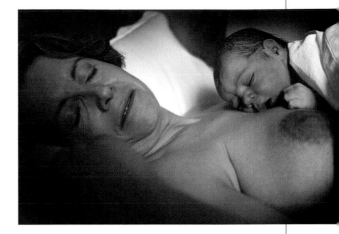

Today in Western countries, mothers are up and about almost immediately showing off their new offsprings to all and sundry, although in some Catholic countries, babies don't usually emerge until they are christened. Throughout Asia, however, mothers and babies still continue to be specially pampered, often with special massages.

One of the hardest aspects of new parenthood is the conflict between wanting to introduce all your friends and family to your new baby and creating vital space and time during which you can settle down together. Only you can be the judge of how to balance this but do not feel guilty about taking every opportunity to sleep and rest. Many of your usual chores can be left for a couple of weeks and the more rested, relaxed, and stress-free as possible you are during those first few weeks, the more likely your baby will be content. Creating one or two visitor-free weeks, only inviting those who are prepared to help with your basic needs, is essential, for these precious early days with your newborn baby can never be recaptured. For those who choose to breastfeed, this day-time rest will be essential, as it provides your body with some regeneration time and helps your milk supply.

A NURTURING ENVIRONMENT

Creating an environment that helps your baby feel safe and secure is very important. Environment in this sense does not mean aesthetic or material belongings, but enabling your baby to have as much close contact with you as possible. If you nurture your newborn intensively from day one, you will dramatically influence the adult that he will become and thus the contribution he is able to make to society throughout his lifetime.

A newborn baby knows nothing of greed, anger or manipulation. Born to survive, he will instinctively demonstrate from the beginning which of his survival needs must be met by crying until those needs are satisfied. Interestingly, most new mothers begin to interpret these cries fairly early. Before you know it, you'll be able to tell whether he's hungry, uncomfortable or bored!

Both you and the baby's father should spend time with him, in skin-to-skin contact. This will give him plenty of reassurance and help to keep him warm.

Sleeping together is another opportunity for bonding. Your baby will feel secure because he can smell his mother and he can feel the warmth of your body next to him. Of course, it is highly discouraged by those in the "routine" business, but it certainly has a very soothing effect on your baby! Even if you simply allow your baby to fall asleep at your breast, this is something all mothers who behave instinctively will feel totally comfortable with.

Although this book is not a guide to the first year, I feel the word "routine" needs to be put into context. To many, this word is associated with getting your baby into a feeding, playing and sleeping pattern that is similar every day and allows you and your baby to develop familiar habits. These days, when most mothers are trying to achieve so much, even a couple of weeks after the arrival of a new baby it is obvious to see the value of a routine. However, I do think it is possible to work with your baby towards a mutually agreed pattern, rather than a prescriptive and imposed routine that often involves training your baby using some rather distressing techniques. I, for one, could never let my baby cry, and if you feel the same way, you have my complete sympathy. But why should you let your baby cry? Your baby is trying to communicate with you in the only way he knows; ignoring that communication or attempting to stifle it with a pacifier sends a very clear message to him. In the early days, a baby needs as much love, comfort and reassurance as you can give. Do not feel that you are spoiling your baby or heading down the path of bad habits. If your instinct tells you to pick up your baby and rock him in your arms until he is asleep, let your instincts guide you. On no account should you feel guilty about overindulging your baby. I applaud your maternal instinct and urge you to continue using it.

By tenderly embracing your newborn, skin to skin, you afford him the ability to touch and smell the only person that he has ever known and provide him with the warmth so important to him as his own heat-regulating mechanism is yet still immature.

Newborn babies are incredibly intelligent for they are born with the ability to communicate their needs. It is you who must gradually learn how to interpret and understand what those needs may be. It is all too easy to become influenced and therefore distracted as you concentrate too hard on training your baby to fit into your lifestyle and our adult world. As a result, you deny your newborn and yourself the essential opportunity to develop a mutually satisfying method of interaction, which in the early days, should have no time constraints.

A newborn baby is defenceless and vulnerable, totally dependent on his carers to provide for all his needs. That said, babies are born with an amazingly strong instinct

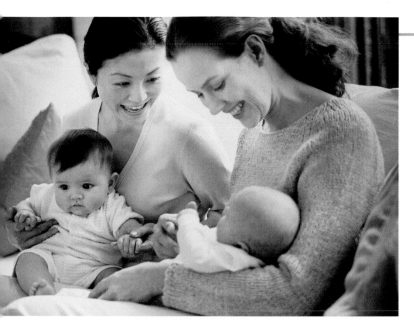

Right from the start, babies begin to exhibit individual personality traits – some more "fussy" than others. But all babies will benefit from continual close attention from their mothers. It is this that makes them more confident individuals, both as babies and as adults.

to survive. That survival is based on three potentially simple needs: food, love and warmth. Food implies not only the satisfaction of hunger, but also the fulfilment of your baby's emotional needs as he is held at your breast to be fed. Love is encapsulated by moments of complete peace and tranquillity, as when you hold your newborn tenderly in your arms, for you are the only person he truly knows and trusts. And warmth is provided by close skin-to-skin contact with your baby, where he can safely maintain his body temperature surrounded by your distinctive smell that is utterly reassuring.

This degree of intensive nurturing allows you, eager to embrace your newborn's every need, to create the beginning of your baby's foundation of emotional security. As you learn to harmonize your maternal instincts with the instinctive demands of your baby, a contented mother and baby will evolve. And a baby that is eager to explore his now and forever external existence.

STRIKING A BALANCE

As with all aspects of parenting, a balance will be struck. Committing all your time to a new baby will gradually be balanced with maintaining the status quo within your family. The first few weeks are challenging. Not only are you getting to know your baby, establishing a feeding pattern and understanding his cries, you are also trying to balance the demands of your household. Your husband, for example, may be starting to doubt his position on your ladder of affections and may need additional reassurance about how you feel, especially if you are not yet feeling ready to resume a sexual relationship. Or, you may have other children who were so excited about the birth of their brother or sister and now are not sure what the reality means for them, especially as the new baby doesn't quite meet their expectations of a permanent playmate. Or it may simply be your house pet who is not getting the "lap time" it previously enjoyed and starts to display some unpredictable behaviour patterns. Every family lives differently together and what may work for one may not be suitable for another. Much of the first few weeks will involve working with the new family member to create a new living environment within which all family members feel comfortable.

Well-intentioned carers will often feel that they are helping by parting a mother from her infant in order that she has a few moments of quality time. But a mother will be unable to rest until she can see and feel her baby safely beside her where, once again, she can take heed of the powerful maternal instinct which ensures her baby's wellbeing both day and night.

Most women are surprised at how enjoyable as well as fulfilling breastfeeding can be. By breastfeeding, not only do you look after your baby's physical need to be nourished but his emotional needs as well.

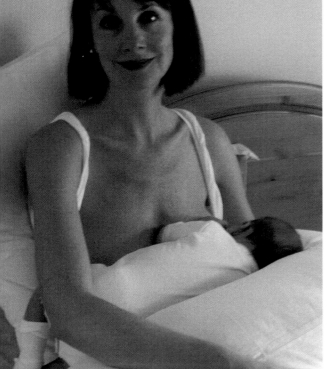

FEEDING

Soon after his birth a baby will display the rooting reflex in his search for food. In the fullness of time and with no barriers between your baby and your breast, he will fix freely and instinctively in order to suckle enthusiastically. The close contact of breastfeeding ensures the growing bond between mother and baby. Nature is very clever in making us spend quality time with our young – breastfeeding cannot be rushed. Breastfeeding has infinite advantages, which are continually being endorsed by sound research. Not least is the mother's passing over to her infant of what is referred to as "passive immunity" – that is, protection against any childhood diseases that the mother has had. The early milk, colostrum, is high and rich in calories, and flows out at exactly the correct temperature.

FREE TO FEED

I recommend that newly delivered mothers enjoy the freedom of loose-fitting clothing and possibly refrain from wearing

*Carol, an American mother who I cared for, told me she had been adamant before becoming pregnant that she was never going to breastfeed. Once pregnant, however, she changed her mind completely, allowing her maternal instincts total freedom. She found to her total fulfilment and to the amazement of her husband, that she really enjoyed breastfeeding. She now has a healthy baby son who is thriving on being fully breastfed.

the seemingly mandatory feeding bra for the first week or two. I also suggest dressing your infant in a minimum of clothing; if clothing is restricted, your newborn baby will be more able to enjoy the close physical contact he has with you and his father. If the temperature permits, try leaving on just his nappy. Research has demonstrated the benefit of prolonged skin-to-skin contact between mother and baby. It encourages good lactation, and a baby becomes more settled as he bathes in the increasing security of his mother's touch and smell. By not wearing a bra until you are more mobile, your nipples, which quite often may become sore from your initial attempts of establishing breastfeeding, benefit not only from air but also the healing powers of breast milk, which can gently be expressed and massaged into to your nipple, especially after feeding. Often, too, newborns have "sticky eyes". This is not an infection but the result of an, as yet, not fully opened tear duct allowing debris to accumulate. A drop or two of breast milk should remedy the problem. Not wearing a bra also prevents your nipples from becoming flattened, adding another possible difficulty to the establishment of breastfeeding. Breast pads, if used too soon after the birth, create the perfect medium for bacteria to survive – sweetness, moisture and warmth. My personal experience is that there have been far fewer cases of mastitis in the many years that I have been advising the initial abandonment of bras. There is no strict time or duration that a mother should refrain from wearing a bra. Your decision will be based on your own personal comfort. But, once your baby becomes increasingly expert at breastfeeding, if you don't wear a bra, he will be able to access your breast quietly and efficiently day or night without difficulty and with least disturbance to you.

So many mothers feel pressured by their own mothers, relatives, friends and society itself, to ignore their strong maternal instincts and desire to keep their newborn babies close to them at all times, completely demand-feeding as and when their babies indicate, thus respecting their babies' own instincts. It is often forgotten that breastfeeding has two overriding advantages to the baby. Firstly, it is his best source of nourishment. His

My own daughter-in-law, Lyndsay, herself incredibly maternal and instinctive having birthed her first-born baby, Megan, struggled to breastfeed while in hospital not only with the mechanics of breastfeeding but more dramatically, with the plethora of well-intentioned but completely conflicting advice. At Lyndsay's request upon her return home, I moved in, keen to support her. The most demanding time, as with most first-time mothers, was during the small hours of the morning. Lyndsay's nipples were very sore, not yet toughened against the intense sucking action of her new baby who was crying and lustily demanding food immediately. After three days and nights of stoic determination by Lindsay, Megan began fixing well at the breast and feeding enthusiastically. Lyndsay could now begin to relax and enjoy her baby daughter to the full, but she confesses that had she not had such support and some help in correct technique, she would have abandoned breastfeeding.

stomach is the size of a walnut, hence the need in the early days and weeks for frequent feeding. Secondly, breastfeeding is also the maximum source of emotional security a mother can provide her child. Safe in your arms, breastfeeding skin-to-skin, you are providing the unique and irreplaceable foundation of emotional security for your newborn baby. The more diluted this incredibly important opportunity for intensive mothering is, the more unsettled your baby will become. He will cry so much more. For your baby crying is the only means of communication and yet in the early days and weeks so easily assuaged through food, love and warmth.

A mother who cannot or does not wish to breastfeed her baby must not be made to feel guilty. However, if the subject is discussed early between mother and midwife, then there will be an opportunity to explore the feelings behind this decision. Many mothers change their minds for many reasons, not least of all, understanding the huge benefits that breastfeeding has.

A mother who is committed, for whatever reason, to formula-feeding must be afforded all the help and support regarding her decision. It is still possible for a formula-feeding mother to simulate the skin-to-skin contact with her newborn, just as if she was breastfeeding. While I am a great advocate of breastfeeding, I fully endorse a mother who has decided that bottle-feeding is the best option for her and her baby. There are advantages to bottle-feeding that cannot be overlooked, such as the ability for the partner to feed the baby and allow the mother to rest, as well as the partner's own ability to bond with their baby.

Establishing a breastfeeding rhythm may not happen immediately. The first few days may be very erratic as your body understands the supply and demand pattern required for its production of milk. The more your baby suckles, the more your breasts will supply. Your breasts may feel very sore and tender and it is quite normal to find breastfeeding more painful than you had anticipated. This should settle down gradually but may take as long as six weeks to establish, and eventually breastfeeding will become a pleasurable activity.

For mothers who desperately want to breastfeed their babies and are unable to do so, this time can be quite distressing, and often one of the earliest challenges of new parenthood. Being a new mother is an emotional time as you deal not only with the demands of your baby but also with the demands of your changing body, heavily influenced by hormonal action. My personal experience has been that there are actually very few cases where a mother really cannot breastfeed her baby but it may require determination, perseverance and a supporting carer who will help you through. A typical example of mothers believing that breastfeeding is impossible is when their babies are premature. Yet there is well-documented, sound research indicating that in such a case it is even more important to afford the baby skin-to-skin contact with his mother, increasing the opportunity for good lactation, and the eventual establishment of breastfeeding.

The subject of feeding has always attracted a host of opinions. There was a decade when breastfeeding was strongly discouraged and the bottle was accepted as the "norm". These days, although there are still diverse views, the vast majority appear to recognize the benefits of breastfeeding. As I have said, it is not just the nutritional value that underpins this argument but also the unquestionable emotional foundation that it provides a baby.

Enjoy your baby in whatever way you like and if this means just holding your baby close and looking into his eyes, I assure you your instincts are flowing!

However, when all is said and done, an important part of feeding is being relaxed. There is no point striving to produce milk and encouraging your baby to suckle if you are not happy and comfortable. Feeding is a time for being together, quietly bonding, and studying each other's faces. If this becomes replaced by anguish and frustration, by considering the options available, even if they conflict with your initial aspirations, you may be able to relax and enjoy your baby which is, after all, the most important part of being a mother.

✳ Julia, pregnant with her third baby and already the mother of two healthy little boys, progressed through pregnancy without complication although with the demands of being a wife and mother and only limited help available, she started to tire easily towards the end of her pregnancy. The birth at home of her third son took place in a candle-lit room, totally naturally, just as she had planned and wanted. With breastfeeding well-established once more, I said farewell at six weeks.

Julia's baby was three-and-a-half months when she telephoned me. An exhausted voice was telling me that she was attempting to encourage her baby to sleep in his crib, whereas up until then he had enjoyed the skin-to-skin contact he'd had with his mother as they shared a bed. Julia was in conflict with her instincts, not really wanting to abandon the close contact she had shared with her baby, but desperate to achieve some quality sleep. Her baby was expressing his needs through his only means of communicating distress – crying until his instinctive need was met. Expressing her breast milk was an option that Julia had already tried without success. She admitted to feeling incredibly guilty about the whole situation. My advice to this apparently exhausted mother was to offer her baby an occasional bottle of formula milk, preferably given by her partner as a night feed, thus affording her the opportunity of some quality sleep. She sounded relieved at being offered an alternative choice.

Two weeks later I met up with Julia. She had bought some bottles and some formula but had not needed to use them. Her baby was still bed-sharing and continued to be the contented little baby he had always been. Julia had been able to acknowledge and respect her instincts, and was now sleeping better and coping with the demands of her family, reassured in the knowledge that her baby son would all too soon become secure and confident like her other two children.

SLEEPING

If you're a new mother, sleep will often become a silent obsession that only those who have had a baby can understand! My advice to new parents is to turn your clocks to the wall so that you are blissfully unaware as to when and for how long your baby has breastfed. Not only is it important that you are well rested and able to replenish your energy levels, but your baby depends on good sleep in order to eat well, grow and develop. A well-rested baby usually makes for a happy baby. Of course, every baby has a different sleep pattern and requirement – just as some adults only need six hours a night and others need ten.

Just as how you feed your baby is a personal and instinctive decision, so, too, is the way you will meet your baby's sleep needs. Bookshop shelves are lined with titles giving advice on how to achieve good sleeping patterns, and the direction you take will depend on your individual beliefs and be dramatically influenced by what is acceptable to you and your partner.

An instinctive mother with her satisfied newborn baby in her arms will, given the opportunity, gently rock her baby until, with heavy eyelids, he gently falls asleep. What better way for a mother to maintain her baby's total feeling of security? Yet mothers are often advised that by rocking their babies to sleep they are spoiling their child and will surely pay for this indulgence in the fullness of time: these are human beings we are talking about, not animals that need to be trained.

The more time you spend with your newborn, the more effort you are putting into creating a long-lasting relationship.

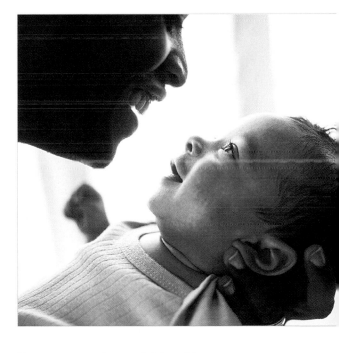

COMFORTING

It is important to recognize that the cry of a newborn baby means something. Parents who spend quality time with their new babies have the opportunity to start getting to know their baby's cries and which needs must be met. Babies do not come armed with emotional blackmail techniques and manipulation skills; they come with basic instincts and a cry that allows them to voice when those needs are not met. By cuddling and rocking your baby you are not developing bad habits that will continue until your child is older; you are developing the essential bond that creates a trusting relationship between you and your child. How many women have said to me: "I would pick my baby up but I read it will become a bad habit." Let me assure you, at two weeks old, your baby is not developing bad habits.

*Lucille's first baby had been very demanding. The hospital birth and labour had not gone well for Lucille and her baby had spent her first night in the special-care baby unit. Establishing breastfeeding took many fretful weeks. When she was pregnant the second time, she became more and more certain she wanted to birth her baby at home. Her husband was less sure, having been quite dramatically affected by his daughter's birth. Lucille eventually birthed her 9 lb son at home, with her husband's support. She was in control throughout her labour and the birth, and she and the baby spent the first week in skin-to-skin contact morning, noon and night, breastfeeding him on demand. With mother and son working harmoniously and instinctively together, there has been little or no crying. He cries only to alert her that he is hungry.

Babies always cry for a reason. Ignoring a cry will interfere with your baby's emotional security. Today's society appears to be obsessed with routine, and babies are very often made to slot into this routine by being given a pacifier. Why? Did nature really mean for our babies' cries, their only means of communication, to be hushed using an aid often held firmly in place by an adult's hand? What are we doing to our babies when we make it impossible for them to communicate their needs?

Jean Liedloff, in her book *The Continuum Concept*, further describes the emotional significance of the immediate days and weeks following the birth of a baby in her chapter on "The Beginning of Life". She talks of expectations that were established within the womb and the flexibility of the newborn to adapt these expectations to his new environment within certain limits. "Every nerve ending under his newly exposed skin craves the expected embrace; all of his being, the character of all he is, leads to his being held in arms. For millions of years newborn babies have been held close to their mothers from the moment of birth ... The state of consciousness of an infant changes enormously during the in-arms phase ... If he feels safe, wanted and 'at home' in the midst of activity before he can think, his view of later experiences will be very distinct in character from those of a child who feels unwelcome, unstimulated by the experiences he has missed and accustomed to living in a state of want, though the later experiences of both may be identical."

The mother who intensively nurtures her newborn for as long as he demonstrates that he needs that level of nurturing, will equip him with such a strong foundation of emotional security that he will remain so as he grows. It all begins from day one and, as we are beginning to appreciate, even earlier. Society should be responsible for supporting new parents by affording them maximum time with their babies. A network of support should relieve new parents of all basic chores, thus affording them precious time in the early days of their baby's life to get to know this new little person. These days can never be recaptured.

DAILY CARE

Observe almost all babies from birth onwards and you will become increasingly aware that their feet hardly ever see the light of day. Almost from the minute they are born, babies are enclosed in baby grows or sleep suits with just their little hands and faces exposed (providing they do not have scratch-mittens!). Today's babies have their sensitive little feet encased in booties, socks, slippers and even trainers, depriving them of the essential opportunity of exploring the different textures and surfaces that their sensitive feet appreciate and need. More importantly, anyone holding a baby whose feet are exposed, will automatically stroke, massage or play with them, almost providing a baby with the most instinctive form of reflexology. Within a few short weeks, the baby will raise his legs so that he, too, will begin to explore his interesting little feet and toes.

Of course, in cold weather a baby needs to be wrapped warmly when venturing outdoors, but once indoors, or when warmer weather appears, it is beneficial to allow your baby's feet the opportunity to breathe and grow without restriction. To a baby, sleeping scratch-mittens are what boxing gloves would be like to an adult. A baby will not inflict so much damage on himself that it could become dangerous. In fact, a baby's little nails do not need to be bitten or cut as unintentional harm can result. It is quite possible to draw blood by cutting too close to the skin and the human mouth is full of bacteria. As they are usually quite soft, most babies' nails will break off naturally when they get to a certain length. If not, picking the sharp corners gently and peeling the nail across the top will suffice.

Following the birth of their babies using a pool, most mothers positively luxuriate in the post-birth inviting warmth of a deep bath shared with their newborns. This, I suggest to the proud parents, should be the first and last time that their new baby is bathed until the cord stump has separated. This separation is achieved by a bacterial process, dry gangrene. In my experience, if the cord is moistened by bathing, not only is the separation process prolonged, but the smell of rotting tissue can be overwhelming.

Imagine the joy once the cord stump has separated. It is then that I suggest the ultimate way of bathing a baby. The parents run a really warm bath and either one or both of them enter the tub with their newborn, allowing the relaxing water to envelope them, often with the mother breastfeeding.

MASTERING PARENTHOOD

Building expectations is a natural process and we all want to be perfect parents. One of the hardest truths to acknowledge as a new parent is that your best is good enough, no matter how far it is from the expectations you set before giving birth. Your best will not always be perfect and your baby will cry. This does not mean you are failing or that you are not a successful parent. It means you and your baby are getting to know each other, you are communicating, and you are learning more and more each day. Nobody makes a perfect parent and nobody has all the answers. Of course you should seek help and look to those around you to give you support and guidance, but you know your baby better than anyone else, and the answers will come sooner or later. Let your instincts guide you and allow yourself time to develop into your new role. As much as parenthood is a natural process, it is also a continuous learning curve. Do not chastise yourself two months into being a parent if life post birth is not as you imagined. Furthermore, do not become stressed by every other person you know who seems to be doing a better job than you. You are doing your best and this is all your baby needs. What is right for another person's baby may not be right for yours, so be prepared to do a little resetting of expectations and adjusting – this is all part of flexible parenting! Above all, maintain your sense of humour. There's usually a funny side to every situation!

You have come a long way in such a short time. The journey has exposed a vulnerability not previously experienced. But nature had equipped you with deep and powerful instincts so you travelled along that path safely, secure in the knowledge that you'd be able to identify when all was not well. Having made that journey, hopefully with a strong feeling of fulfilment, your baby having completed what some people describe as the most potentially hazardous trip of a lifetime, you are ready now to continue down the path of life together.

Becoming a parent can, for some, appear to be a daunting prospect. It is a huge responsibility and involves a commitment that each one of us strives to fulfil the best we can. Just as with pregnancy and birth, your reawakened instincts are there to guide you – trust them. Respect your child for he, too, is a unique individual. Love your child and let him know that he is loved. Be a friend to your child and listen to what he has to say, for children are wise and see life from a totally different perspective from adults. With flexible parental guidance, influenced by your own beliefs, you will go forward with increasing confidence. Trust yourself, for there is no rule book. We all strive to be the best parents – our best is all we can do.

BIBLIOGRAPHY

Professor Robert Winston
Human Instinct, Bantam Press, 2002

Dr Christiane Northrup
Women's Bodies Women's Wisdom, Bantam Dell, 2002

Sheila Kitzinger
Rediscovering Birth, Simon & Schuster, 2001

Michel Odent
Birth Reborn, Birth Works, 1994

Dr Thomas Verny with John Kelly
The Secret Life of the Unborn Child, Time Warner, 1988

Pat Thomas
Alternative Therapies for Pregnancy & Birth, Vega, 2002

Jean Liedloff
The Continuum Concept, Arkana, 1989

SUGGESTED FURTHER READING

Janet Balaskas & Yehudi Gordon
The Encyclopaedia of Pregnancy & Birth, Little Brown, 1989

Elisabeth Hallett
Stories of the Unborn Soul, Writer's Club Press, 2001

Tracy Hogg with Melinda Blau
Secrets of the Baby Whisperer, Vermillion, 2001

Sue Gerhardt **Why Love Matters,** Brunner-Routledge, 2004

RECOMMENDED WEBSITES

www.aims.org.uk
www.birthchoiceuk.com
www.infochoice.org
www.gentlebirth.org
www.homebirth.org.uk
www.activebirthcentre.com
www.nctpregnancyandbabycare.com

CARROLL & BROWN WOULD LIKE TO THANK:

All the parents and babies who kindly allowed us to print their birth photographs.

Production Karol Davies
Computer Management Paul Stradling
Proofreader Geoffrey West
Picture Researcher Sandra Schneider

PICTURE CREDITS

Corbis p56 (The Cover Story), p59 (Jules Perrier);
Getty Images p27, 50, 54, 73, 96, 99, 108, 111, 119;
Mother and Baby Picture Library p115 (Ruth Jenkinson);
Science Photo Library p10 (Hattie Young), p31 (Sidney Moulds), p35 (Larry Mulvehill), p42 (S. Davidson, Custom Medical Stock Photo), p89 (Ian Hooton), p120 (Hans-Ulrich Osterwalder), p131 (Heny Allis), p135 (Ron Reid), p141 (Hattie Young).